Systems Thinking
for Health Organizations, Leadership, and Policy

Think Globally, Act Locally

James A. Johnson, PhD, MSc, MPA
Douglas E. Anderson, DHA, FACHE

Copyright © 2017 by James A. Johnson and Douglas E. Anderson

Sentia Publishing Company has the exclusive rights to reproduce this work, to prepare derivative works from this work, to publicly distribute this work, to publicly perform this work, and to publicly display this work.

All rights reserved. No part of this publication may be reproduced, stored in a retrieval system, or transmitted, in any form or by any means, electronic, mechanical, photocopying, recording, or otherwise, without the prior written permission of the copyright owner.

Printed in the United States of America
ISBN 978-0-9987874-6-6

Table of Contents

Preface vii
How to Use this Book viii
PART I: FOUNDATIONS 1
   Chapter 1: Systems Thinking For Health 3
   Chapter 2: Associated Theories of Systems Thinking 12
   Chapter 3: The Health System as a "System of Systems" 21
   Chapter 4: Levels of Integration in Complex Adaptive Health Systems 26
PART II: METHODS AND TOOLS 39
   Chapter 5: Identification of the Characteristics and Concepts of Complex Systems .. 41
   Chapter 7: Fundamental Tools – Stocks, Flows, and Loops 55
Part III: APPLICATIONS 99
   Chapter 10: Understanding Frames of Reference in the Context of a Opioid Crisis . 101
   Chapter 11: Ending Homelessness --- Stock-n-Flow and Causal Loop Diagrams 109
   Chapter 12: Using Causal Loops to Reduce Neonatal Mortality in Uganda 117
PART IV: MOVING FORWARD 123
   Chapter 14: Need for Global Health Systems Leadership 126
   Chapter 15: Integration of Systems Thinking with Strategic Planning 132
   Chapter 16: A Quadruple Aim: Integrated Community Health System Model 135
   Chapter 17: Countering Pathological Archetypes to Improve High Reliability Healthcare 142
   Chapter 18: Epilogue – Leader Development to Think Globally and Act Locally 148
Appendix 153
About the Authors 155
References 157
Index 167

List of Figures

PART I

PART 1, CHAPTER 1, FIGURE 1: HUMAN BODY AS A LIVING SYSTEM OF SYSTEMS 7

PART 1, CHAPTER 2, FIGURE 2: ENGELS MODEL 14

PART 1, CHAPTER 3, FIGURE 3: HEALTH SYSTEM AS A SET OF INPUTS-PROCESSES-OUTPUTS 22

PART 1, CHAPTER 4, FIGURE 4: BASIC CRITICAL THINKING MODEL 28

PART 1, CHAPTER 4, FIGURE 5: SIMPLE CAUSAL FEEDBACK LOOP DIAGRAM 29

PART 1, CHAPTER 4, FIGURE 6: EXAMPLE OF FEEDBACK LOOP USING BUILDING HEALTHIER COMMUNITIES AS AN EXAMPLE. 31

PART II

PART 2, CHAPTER 5, FIGURE 7: EVENTS, PATTERNS, AND STRUCTURE 42

PART 2, CHAPTER 7, FIGURE 8: HUMANISTIC BUILDING BLOCK FOR SYSTEMS THINKING 56

PART 2, CHAPTER 7, FIGURE 9: HUMANISTIC SYSTEMS THINKING MODEL TO ILLUSTRATE SYSTEMS THINKING 57

PART 2, CHAPTER 7, FIGURE 10: SIMPLE INPUT, PROCESS, AND OUTPUT MODEL ILLUSTRATING STOCKS, FLOWS, AND RATES 59

PART 2, CHAPTER 7, FIGURE 11: ILLUSTRATION OF CAUSAL LINKS AS PART OF STOCKS, FLOWS, AND RATES 60

PART 2, CHAPTER 7, FIGURE 12: CIRCULAR THINKING VERSUS LINEAR THINKING IN SYSTEMS THINKING 61

PART 2, CHAPTER 7, FIGURE 13: ILLUSTRATION OF CAUSAL LINKS AND LOOPS BETWEEN HUMAN FUNCTIONS AND THINKING 62

PART 2, CHAPTER 8, FIGURE 14: UNDERSTANDING HOW TO CREATE HEALTHIER COMMUNITIES. ADAPTED BY JOHNSON AND ANDERSON FROM MILSTEIN, B, OVERVIEW OF SYSTEMS DYNAMICS SIMULATION MODELING, SYSTEMS THINKING AND MODELING WORKSHOP; 66

PART 2, CHAPTER 8, FIGURE 15: HOW THE HEALTH SYSTEM SHOULD WORK USING POLICY INTERVENTION AND LEVERAGE POINTS. UNDERSTANDING HOW TO CREATE HEALTHIER COMMUNITIES. 67

PART 2, CHAPTER 8, FIGURE 16: LINEAR VERSUS SYSTEMS THINKING AND DECISION-MAKING. 69

PART 2, CHAPTER 8, FIGURE 17: ILLUSTRATION ON HOW CAUSAL LOOP DIAGRAMS ARE USED FOR MAPPING STROKE CARE PROCESSES. 73

PART 2, CHAPTER 9, FIGURE 18: ILLUSTRATION OF THE TYPICAL ARCHETYPE AND REINFORCING OR BALANCING LOOPS 78

PART III

PART 3, CHAPTER 11, FIGURE 19: SOCIAL DETERMINANTS OF HEALTH IN RELATION TO HOMELESSNESS AS ADOPTED BY HEALTHY PEOPLE 2020, FROM THE CENTER FOR DISEASE AND PREVENTION (CDC) 109

PART 3, CHAPTER 11, FIGURE 20: ILLUSTRATION OF STAGES OF HOMELESSNESS WITH STOCK AND FLOW RATES OR LEVERAGE POINTS FOR POLICY INTERVENTION. 112

PART 3, CHAPTER 11, FIGURE 21: BALANCING AND REINFORCING LOOPS TO ILLUSTRATE HOMELESSNESS IN A TYPICAL COMMUNITY. 114

PART 3, CHAPTER 11, FIGURE 22: APPLYING COLLABORATION AND COMMUNICATION TO MAKE DECISIONS AT KEY STOCK AND FLOW POINTS. 115

PART 3, CHAPTER 12, FIGURE 23: INITIAL PLANNING FOR SYSTEMS THINKING CASE IN UGANDA. 117

PART 3, CHAPTER 12, FIGURE 24: ILLUSTRATION OF BALANCING AND REINFORCING LOOPS.

PART 3, CHAPTER 12, FIGURE 25: AGENT MODELING MAPPING MODEL AND SYSTEMS DYNAMICS. 120

PART 3, CHAPTER 12, FIGURE 26: USE OF CAUSAL LOOPS DIAGRAMS TO CREATE SUSTAINABLE SOLUTIONS. 121

PART IV

PART 4, CHAPTER 16, FIGURE 27: THE QUADRUPLE AIM. INTEGRATING THE TRIPLE AIM AND SOCIAL DETERMINANTS OF HEALTH 138

List Of Tables

Number	Title	Page
1	Health Systems Building Blocks (Critical Success Factors)	30
2	Methods, Models, and Tools	49
3	Applications, Actions, Actors and Stakeholder Opioids Crisis	103

Preface

In an era of a dynamic, uncertain, complex, and ambiguous health challenges at all levels and in every setting, *Systems Thinking for Health: Organizations, Leadership, and Policy* is long overdue. Popularized in the 1960's and then again in the 1990s, systems thinking principles and theories have waxed and waned in the management sciences, while retaining saliency in engineering and the biological sciences. Now, "Systems Thinking" has gained wider acceptance and applicability in the medical social sciences, especially in the domains of global and public health. we wrote this book to elevate and illustrate the potential for health systems transformation and sustainability. Systems thinking challenges health leaders and professionals to assess the interactions and interdependencies among elements (often competing) in a system, then seek out opportunities to generate sustainable solutions.

Why take the time to read this book? Fundamentally, this book explores the question of what and how systems thinking adds to the field of healthcare, public health, policy, and global while also improving health leader effectiveness. Systems thinking will help you and others discover hidden assumptions, drive bolder thinking, and express problems or ideas in a global manner. By picking up this book, you have taken the first step in learning how to use a powerful array of systems thinking tools. Systems thinking focuses on non-linear assumptions about human behavior and feedback loops to determine a system's behavior over time to find leverage points to create the most reliable and innovative health systems that are sustainable with a goal of better health for all. The methods and tools presented in this book are suited for different types of inquiry and different health settings and levels. Furthermore, we describe the foundations of systems thinking, while providing methods, tools and applications to enhance the reader's understanding and utility of such an approach and worldview. Systems thinking offers a valuable approach to addressing the most persistent organizational, community, and global challenges we face today and tomorrow.

This is the first comprehensive book to provide a systems thinking perspective to focus exclusively on health. By incorporating theories, concepts, applications, case studies, and possibilities, we have also provided a practical book to enhance one's own leadership capabilities. Systems thinking has a power and emergent potential that is hard to resist once it is understood. We hope to help strengthen our global health network and facilitate the formation of a community of practice where health professionals interested in applying systems thinking and complexity theory can share and learn together. The subtitle of this book is one you are certain to already be familiar with, *"Think Globally, Act Locally"*. We anticipate, with the material presented here, you will now be able to do so more effectively, systemically, and holistically.

Enjoy this exciting learning journey you are about to embark upon!

~ *James A. Johnson*   ~ *Douglas E. Anderson*

How to Use this Book

The competency of systems thinking, as presented in this book, marks a dramatic shift from the linear or reductionist and analytic way of thinking for several reasons. First, this book provides a foundation (or refresher) for systems thinking utilizes levels of analysis and tools from the micro (individual) to the macro (global) in the context of numerous health settings. We explain fundamental concepts, methods, and tools. Examples and case studies presented throughout on health leadership, organizations, and policy challenges illustrate the importance of systems thinking.

Second, the book introduces or perhaps reintroduces systems thinking as a promising approach to addressing today's and tomorrow's complex health challenges. Because systems themselves are so complex and interconnected with everything around them, it is also impossible to see the entire system on paper. For this reason, the tools and case studies are meant to offer illustrative examples and possibilities related to health systems dynamics, behaviors, and dysfunctions.

Third, our pledge to the reader is to convey the often abstract characteristics of systems thinking and translate them into practical examples for health leaders may so they may generate systemic and sustainable solutions. Health systems research, policy, and theories are constantly evolving to include systems thinking skills. For example, health-related case studies continue to emerge, serving to facilitate the integration of community health and health care systems or sustainment of fragile international health systems development..

Finally, readers are urged to view the book as a learning journey. Understanding and application of systems thinking are presented in four parts: Introduction, Methods and Tools, Applications, and Moving Forward. These parts provide a "building block" approach to enhance understanding of how systems thinking can solve complex, ongoing, and chronic or wicked health systems problems. These problems must be solved by collaboration within or outside the walls of the organization as a whole systems approach to building innovative and reliable health systems and healthier populations at any level. Systems thinking will facilitate much needed collaboration.

Structure of the Primer

The reader's learning journey throughout the book creates a foundation for systems thinking and the characteristics of systems, while also providing definitions of systems thinking, methods and tools, providing applications and challenging readers to think about the potential and possibilities.

Part I is organized in a way to provide a foundation (or refresher) for systems thinking by utilizing levels of analysis from the micro (individual) to the macro (global). Part I also provides the motivation for discussing the importance of systems thinking today. The primer reviews the origins of systems thinking, describing a range of the theories, methods, and tools.

Part II provides an overview of concepts, methods, and tools for systems thinking with several illustrations and vignettes. These tools offer a fresh, highly effective way to grasp the complexity of organizational life and to address the stubborn problems that often confront us in organizations of all kinds. For example, systems thinking basics: from concepts to casual loops is designed to help readers discover the principles of systems dynamics and systems thinking and begin using systems thinking tools: behavior over time graphs, causal loop diagrams, uncovering and preventing organization dysfunctions.

Part III reinforces the power of systems thinking with applications, and cases for health leaders, organizations, and policy in the public, private, and nonprofit sectors. These cases challenge readers to embrace the principles of the Institute for Health Improvement's (IHI) Triple Aim and the Centers for Disease and Prevention's (CDC) Social Determinants of Health as a framework for solving complex, ongoing, chronic, or wicked problems plaguing communities at any level.

Part IV challenges leaders and students about aspirations, potential, and possibilities of solving complex and sometimes "wicked" problems with systems thinking. In the spirit of systems thinking, the book is wide-ranging in scope in the context of healthcare, while maintaining a simple elegance in its usability. It is most appropriate for courses in health administration, public health, health policy, global health, and organization development.

The four-part "building block" discussion serves as an introduction to health systems dynamics and thinking. The Appendix provides a set of discussion questions. The book concludes by emphasizing specific models used in systems thinking to provide new opportunities to understand and continuously test and revise our understanding of the nature of things, including how to intervene to improve a population's health at any level.

PART I: FOUNDATIONS

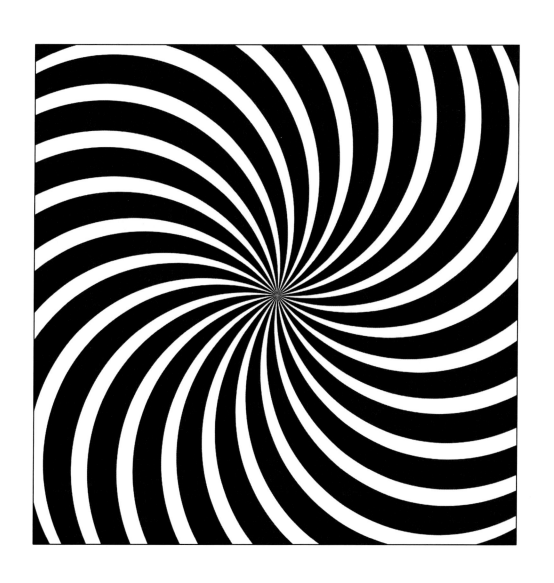

Overview of PART I

PART I challenges health leaders to better understand systems thinking for health by summarizing the essence of its principles, providing an analogy of the human body as a system, illustrating why applying systems thinking is beneficial, and lastly by introducing a range of ideas for the reader to contemplate. It summarizes the dynamic, uncertain, complex, and ambiguous health system at any level and in any setting. Systems thinking challenges health leaders to assess the interdependencies among elements or components within a system, then seek out opportunities to generate sustainable solutions.

Systems thinking will help heath leaders and others discover hidden assumptions, drive bolder thinking, and express problems or ideas from a more global perspective. Gaining an appreciation of systems thinking and associated theories provides the foundation for application.

The complexity of the entire health system and its role within a national and global system should be embraced. Thus, health system improvement and strengthening must be approached in a different way and from a different point of view. This begins with viewing current fragmented health systems around the world as complex adaptive heath systems and then working toward integration and ultimately an interconnected global system of health and well-being for all. The levels and need for integration of health systems is discussed in the context of understanding interdependence, networks of networks and systems of systems, and the enormous number of independent stakeholders and interests, layered within the organization, community, state, and national levels.

Systems thinking necessitates non-linear assumptions and feedback loops to determine a system's behavior over time and find leverage points aimed at creating the most reliable and sustainable health systems If the system is approached by deconstructing the elements of the system, designing how each element should function, and reconstituting the overall system, effective solutions will not be generated. The methods and tools are suited to different types of inquiry and different health settings and levels. In doing so, we describe the foundations of systems thinking, while providing methods, tools and applications to enhance the reader's understanding. Systems thinking offers a valuable emerging perspective on the most persistent organizational and community challenges and your leadership role in their sustainable solutions.

Chapter 1: Systems Thinking For Health

Introflection

Health organizations and health systems operate in an increasingly dynamic, uncertain, complex, and ambiguous environment. There is a dire need to increase and integrate these organization's capabilities so communities at any level anywhere can make effective decisions and engage in behaviors to promulgate the healthiest populations in the world. Perhaps a good starting point in this discussion is to briefly explore the distinction between a system and systems thinking. David Peter Stroh, an applied systemologist who previously worked on projects for the Center for Disease Control and Prevention (CDC) draws on the work of award-winning systems thinker Donella Meadows who defined as system as, "an interconnected set of elements coherently organized in a way to achieve something." Stroh builds on her definition to define systems thinking as "the ability to understand these interconnections in such a way as to achieve a desired purpose."[13] Systems thinking is an effective approach to help organizations, communities, and nations make sense of the myriad interconnectedness and interdependencies of today's health systems. Systems thinking has the potential to produce sustainable solutions to many of the most daunting health challenges we are facing in the world today. Unfortunately, systems thinking as a competency is not sufficiently known nor embraced in health settings and across communities. This chapter challenges health leaders to better understand systems thinking for health by summarizing the essence of its principles, providing an analogy of the human body as a system, illustrating why applying systems thinking is beneficial, and lastly by introducing a range of ideas for the reader to contemplate.

The following quotes from scholars at the vanguard of systems thinking theory and practice underscore the timely relevance of the book you are about to read.

"My own experience suggests that we can forgo the despair created by such common organizational events as change, chaos, information overload, and entrenched behaviors if we recognize that organizations are living systems, possessing the same capacity to adapt and grow that is common to all life."
-Margaret J. Wheatley, *Leadership and the New Science*[14]

"…using the language of systems theory, health organizations can be viewed as complex adaptive systems. Health care is complex in that it is composed of multiple, diverse, interconnected elements, and it is adaptive in that the system is capable of changing and learning from experience and its' environment."
-James A. Johnson, *Health Organizations, 2nd ed.*[15]

"There are four revolutions currently underway that will transform health and health systems. These are the revolutions in: a) life sciences; b) information and communications; c) social justice and equity; and d) systems thinking to transcend complexity.
-Julio Frenk, *Address to the World Health Organization*[16]

What Is Systems Thinking?

Systems thinking is a set of tools and a way of thinking involving an emerging language. In systems thinking, leaders and policy makers look at the whole system rather than its individual parts. They become expansive and non-linear in thinking rather than reductionist and linear. By looking at the whole, leaders are more capable of seeing interrelationships and patterns over time. They begin to understand that problems may be clues or symptomatic of deeper issues within a system or system of systems. Systems thinking challenges health professionals, leaders, and policy makers to look for root causes, bottlenecks, and constraints in ways that allow sustainable solutions to emerge. By doing so, leaders move away from assigning blame and focus on desired outcomes.

Furthermore, systems thinking is proactive, open and circular in nature, as opposed to linear thinking, which tends to be reactive. Systems thinking, despite the technical sounding terms, has three fundamental processes: reinforcing feedback, balancing feedback, and delays. Reinforcing or amplifying feedback loops drive growth or create a decline in system performance at any level. They either spiral up or down. They rarely occur in isolation within a system (team, organization, or community). There are limits to growth and decline, many of which can become dysfunctional especially if organizations are seeking the wrong goals. For example, reinforcing loops can generate an organization's daily patient visit schedule, then several actions such as financial incentives influence growth to certain limits. However, a loop can move in either a positive direction or a negative direction depending on capacity, quality of interactions in a system, experience of care, and policies aimed at creating health versus episodic visits or the desired goal.

Systems Thinking in the Context of Health

In the rapidly changing domains of public health and healthcare delivery systems throughout the world, systems thinking may be viewed as offering valuable insights for understanding and action. The World Health Organization (WHO) describes systems thinking as "an approach to problem solving that views 'problems' as part of a wider, dynamic system. Systems thinking involves much more than a reaction to present outcomes or events. It demands a deeper understanding of the linkages, relationships, interactions, and behaviors among the elements to characterize the entire system."[16]

Because health challenges are complex, solutions will differ depending on individual, time and place, imposing top-down plans of actions will not consistently achieve predictable, positive results. Today, many leaders are trained in machine-age, production thinking, reductionist approach. This method no longer works well. Individual parts do not equate to the system as a whole, especially when the dynamic nature of the external environment affects any of the parts. Some health leaders see systems thinking as a set of powerful tools to facilitate communication and creativity to investigate complex issues. Unfortunately, too many are confused by the amorphous body of theories, methods, and tools involved.

Systems thinking is actually simple but too infrequently applied, particularly in the context of the significant and often chronic problems currently facing the world. Today, systems thinking has the potential to facilitate environments where local individuals, organizations, and communities self-organize to improve health and produce sustainable solutions together. Such approaches can lead to innovative, beneficial results health planners have only imagined. Systems thinking provides frameworks, principles, and approaches to rethink basic assumptions about health, increase local capacity, and unite communities to create high-reliability organizations and healthier populations to increase better health outcomes, productivity, and quality of life. However, if health leaders aim to generate sustainable solutions, embracing systems thinking is a "must do, can't fail" proposition. Systems thinking for health leaders is not overly complicated for several reasons.

First, systems thinking reframes conversations to help others see "whole" systems not "stovepiped" parts in isolation at any level. Systems thinking challenges leaders to identify patterns, interrelationships, and boundaries beyond the issue of the moment, static problems, a department, and organization. Complex, ongoing, and chronic problems such as preventable deaths require a systems approach to reducing harm by changing an organization's culture to create high-reliability health organizations similar to how the airline industry has reduced accidents.

Second, viewing the problem as a whole system in a larger context does not favor breaking problems down into small pieces. Systems thinking prompts investigation and systemic assessment, so complex challenges are assessed through the "viewpoints" of all stakeholders. Systems thinking urges leaders to connect with and mobilize others as a team to recognize and exploit interconnected points resulting in sustainable solutions. For example, ending homelessness has interconnected medical, behavioral, public health, social viewpoints, and solutions. Systems thinking helps stakeholders see the impact of dysfunctional patterns and interactions of their "stovepipes" or "silos" on the system as a whole.

Third, systems thinking is a transformational way of understanding and approaching community based solutions. By seeing the trends, interactions and connections at the individual, team, organization, community, or policy levels leaders more fully understand the need for systemic approaches to solving problems rather than generating solutions in isolation. For example, leaders in health organizations need to understand how social determinants of health, including community culture and demographics affect the volume of services, capacities, and outcomes. Conversely, public health practitioners should understand how the population health component of the Triple Aim could support an initiative within the SDH framework. For example, solving community-level substance abuse problems requires a community-wide approach to integrating health and other organizations to resolving the problem of reducing substance abuse. Furthermore, systems thinking provides a "safe psychological bridge" to view problem situations, allowing for the questioning of hidden assumptions and biases to search for sustainable solutions for community health and non-health systems.

Finally, systems analysis examines the organization through the use of the systems approach. It is a way to address that which impedes or improves an organization and helps create an organization that is healthy. The systems approach to intervention requires leaders to view problems within an organization and examine all of the interactions and interrelations connected with those issues within and outside the organization. For example, the growth and change in any one part of a system affect every other part of the system, when using the systems approach to intervention, one must look at all of the pieces of the whole.

Human Body Analogy

People live and work within systems, while at the same time, people are systems. For example, as described by James Johnson in the recent book *Comparative Health Systems.*

> "The human body is a system composed of many physiological subsystems that are interconnected in a holistic way. The subsystems, including respiratory, circulatory, neurological, endocrine, and musculoskeletal system, communicate and are interdependent. They work together for the purposes of survival, adaptation, growth, and development. They interact with the environment and respond to feedback from within and outside the system. In many ways, the interconnectivity of the various subsystems and it's extension as a whole into the environment form the building blocks of larger systems, such as family, community, and nation."[17]

The figure below illustrates the body and systems thinking analogy. As a whole, the human organism is a system as a whole: a body with a head, a trunk, two arms, two legs, feet, hands, and so on. Some of these systems are living and thinking, and some are not living and thinking. They can be broken down into smaller parts. If we break the body down further, we find the body is comprised of smaller systems: skin, brain, eyes, lungs, liver, stomach, kidney, heart, veins, etc. These smaller systems are comprised of even smaller system elements. The eyes, for example, consist of the cornea, the lens, the iris, the pupil, the sclera, the retina, and optic nerves, among other things.[18] Each of these components is comprised of even smaller systems such as cells and cells themselves are comprised of the membranes, cytoplasm, mitochondria, vacuoles, ribosomes, nuclei, and Golgi bodies.[18] The breakdown of the human body into its smaller systems signifies the system hierarchy.[19]

The Human Body is a System of Parts With Inputs and Outputs	Human Are Complex Adaptive and Sometimes Fragile "Systems of Systems"
Cardiovascular / Circulatory	Interdependent
Integumentary / Exocrine	Interrelated
Lymphatic / Immune	Integrated
Digestive / Excretory	Creative
Muscular / Skeletal	Sensing
Endocrine	Social
Nervous	Feeling
Respiratory	Resilient
Reproductive	Innovative
Renal / Urinary	

Optimal Human Performance Depends on Quality and Quantity of Energy Inputs and Outputs and Environment

Part 1, Chapter 1, Figure 1: Human Body as a Living System of Systems; created by D. Anderson

Health professionals across the full spectrum of health organizations naturally understand living and thinking systems: they deal with living thinking systems every day: human beings. Only thinking systems like humans can want to be healthy and to live a long time, and yet eat themselves to 300 pounds, smoke cigarettes, drink soda, and avoid exercise. However, health professionals need to think beyond the patient, provider, and healthcare team perspective. A system as an entity maintains its existence through the mutual interaction of its parts. The definition describes a family, an operating room (OR), a hospital, nursing home, public health department, or ministry of health for a country and what physicians treat every day – humans.

Health professionals may not go far enough with respect the levels of systems outside their sphere of influence. For example, healthcare professionals typically deal with three different types of systems: clinical, community, and administrative in unknowingly or fragmented ways. What is often missing is a discussion about the kinds, levels, and dysfunctions/functions of systems. In the human body's case, override, or precedence of systems and subsystems is work in motion. All human and health systems are parts of larger systems or levels. The kidney is a part – a subsystem – of the larger body and organ system. The body is part of a larger system called a family. The family, a group of thinking systems, is part of a community, which is a part of the nation. A nation is one part of the group of nations on the planet Earth. Earth itself is a part, a subsystem, of the solar system, and so on.[19]

The human body in action illustrates the systems, subsystems, and levels of systems:

1. Brain to muscles: A human is in a race. The humans run faster and harder.
2. Muscles to brain: The brain transmits what's going on.
3. Brain to Heart: The brain says pump faster and harder. The muscles need more blood flow so the human can win this race.
4. Heart to brain: Okay, but tell the lazy liver to get off its rear and make more energy. Also, tell the lungs we need more oxygen and less carbon dioxide.
5. Brain to the liver: The brain tells the liver to work harder. The human body needs more energy. The muscles produce lactic acid and need the human to flush it out.
6. Liver to brain: The liver obliges and uses stored, previously prepared energy. The liver sends it to the muscles. However, eventually, the human needs to start eating to create energy.
7. Intestines (including the mouth) to brain: Intestines resist eating. The brain knows the body cannot run fast on a full stomach, but another part of the brain overrides it.
8. Liver to intestines (side conversation): The liver acknowledges the situation, but if the race is long, more energy is needed. If the body does not eat the muscles will weaken and convert the pieces into packets of energy.
9. Liver to heart: The heart needs lots of energy, and the liver knows it, but the effects could be overproduction eventually turning into fat.
10. Muscles to all: The muscle says thanks and the human body goes faster and eventually wins.[19]

The examples above represent a system where the parts interact and where there is feedback. The patient and provider interact. The patient and healthcare team interact. The patient eventually has to interact with their families, insurers, another healthcare system such as rehabilitation, and environment as part of the healing process or preventive care plan. When something goes wrong, the provider must find which part of the human is sick and determine why or what part of the system is not helping the patient. Then together, the provider and health teams fix the patient.[19]

In many respects, health professionals, are natural systems thinkers, in that they are typically aware that any "fix" of one part will affect other parts of the system in addition to the one that became ill or injured. Suppose the body parts did not interact and there was no feedback. Now suppose the body is in a swimming race, and the brain decided the body would go faster if it stopped breaking the water every few seconds by raising and lowering the head. What happens when, with no feedback, the brain fails to learn the body has run out of the air? Patient care is a system, where interactions are often in one direction, and there is no effective feedback. Within the parts of the healthcare system, particularly in the policy level, there is no consensus on desired goals or outcomes. The fact health professionals believe anything calls itself a system is systematic; however, the system and subsystems tend to produce perverse incentives and vicious cycles or feedback loops of poor health, access, and outcomes. This is why it is important to apply systems thinking at all levels of the health system.[20,19]

Health Systems Benefits

Systems thinking includes concepts and skills. Health systems thrive on interrelated and interconnected processes, yet few are treated as such. Health professionals understand the interdependence of systems within the human body. For example, they know the respiratory system is made up of many parts and when a patient or cohort of patients has difficulty breathing the entire system must be examined to determine the true cause of the problem. However, if only the presenting problem is addressed (a stuffy nose), they may overlook the true issue (a sinus infection) or cause unintended consequences (prescribing a medication causes the patient to have an allergic reaction). Systems thinking implies parts of a given system – human being, team, organization, or health system – are interdependent and interconnected. An alteration, loss, missed or overlooked information or breakdown of any part affects the function of the whole at any level – patient, team, organization, or community.

From a human and health systems perspective, successful sustainable health systems are integrated as well as within the larger or integrated levels of systems of which they are a part. For a public health system, the social determinants of health provide a framework for well functioning systems.

With the social determinants of health (SDH), discussed in more detail later in this book, combinations of debilitating factors influence individual health, the delivery of health, and community health as a whole. Today, these factors have become increasingly sophisticated and epidemic-like, yet approaches to solving these problems remain problematic. For example, healthcare, public health, and community leaders have struggled to reduce the second and third order effects of obesity, diabetes, poverty, prescription medication abuse, and heart disease. These problems, are multi-faceted, dynamic, and interconnected "wicked problems" because they are chronic, resistant, have multiple causes, and different solutions. Unfortunately, healthcare teams tend to focus on curing individuals within their organizations in the context of the Triple Aim while public health practitioners apply strategies inherent in the social determinants of health, yet neither fully understand how an individual's environment, behaviors, choices affect well-being. Furthermore, when addressing health challenges, policies such as transitioning from volume to value-based reimbursement has maximum impact on both systems while minimizing unintended consequences.

Success with the eradication of smallpox, treatment of diarrhea with oral rehydration solutions, and organ transplants are examples of systems thinking in action. Today's health dilemmas are complex and interdependent at successive levels, rendering cookie cutter approaches to policy development or program implementation in has proven to be inadequate. Obesity, for example, is caused by multiple interacting factors including family history, socioeconomic status, lifestyle, diet, exercise habits, and culture. Healthcare support, procedures, and medications alone won't work. A community approach must be taken including healthier choices at eating and grocery establishments, healthier school lunches, walking, riding, and running paths, and social marketing campaigns. Unfortunately, fragmented approaches, many of which shift the burden onto the healthcare system for quick fixes, results in unintended consequences, such as dependencies, inefficiencies, and inequities.

Systems thinking provides rigorous ways for aligning stakeholders, purpose, process, and expected behaviors to drive solution development beyond the walls of "stovepiped" organizations. Health organizations engaging in systems thinking are able to accomplish the following more effectively:

- *Develop new ways of looking at old problems.*
- *Integrate new information more easily.*
- *See interrelationships and cause and effect more clearly.*
- *Develop patience with implementing change and tolerating implementation or policy delays.*
- *Step away from the blame game and move toward shared responsibility.*
- *See the whole rather than the parts.*

Organizations, like biological systems, are interconnected and have interrelated and interdependent parts that make up the whole. They are living systems that rely on feedback to self-correct. A systems approach sees the organization as a complete system where even small activities, interventions, or changes have an effect on other sub-systems and the organization as a whole. The challenges in today's health system and any potential transformation are abundant. Specific examples include:

- Conceptualization or "ideation" of a new service or next generation product and integration of systems thinking into the organization's strategic planning.
- Reducing preventive harm and deaths by applying systems thinking to create high-reliability healthcare organizations
- Ongoing chronic problems specific populations or cohorts whose health literacy, adherence to medications, or familiarity with the health organization are low.
- Challenges of engaging the community to address a comprehensive approach to reducing homelessness, tobacco cessation, and prescription drug abuse.
- Development of policies and procedures to incentivize the delivery of health versus the production of health through the entire episode of a patient's care.
- Drive strategies to embrace "disruptive" technologies or innovation such as medication drone delivery, vaccine spray or contraception vending machines.
- Building healthier communities such as walking paths, tobacco-free city blocks, and healthy school lunches to improve the quality of life and more productivity.

The most successful health leaders, health professionals, and policy-makers see the big picture; they are constantly seeking to see underlying trends, patterns and possible consequences of actions. They are aware of the larger environmental context such as how a project impacts parts of the system or culture. For some, this ability comes naturally but is not always easy. It is hard to translate systems thinking for others. Systems thinking formalizes analytic processes to provide a method for gaining insight into the underlying system dynamics. Systems thinking provides methods and tools to embrace complexity, recognize interrelations of the parts, see patterns of behavior over time, and generate sustainable solutions.

Reflection

It is often said, humans are creatures of habit, sometimes finding it difficult to recognize counterproductive patterns of behavior. Systems thinking offers perspectives, tools, and processes to enable leaders and organizations to recognize patterns and connections, leading to greater productivity, healthier outcomes, and improved quality of life. The benefits of systems thinking have the potential to solve complex problems by bringing a consistent, big-picture view to all actors and stakeholders focusing on the prioritized value needs of a more complete solution.

Systems thinking addresses recurring problems such as changing expectations, clearer early-stage service or product conception and design, and integrating multiple stakeholder viewpoints or perspectives throughout the process. The result is a shared understanding of the overall problem and the solution purpose, establishment of value-driven priorities across the organization, community, or larger health system. Additionally, it can be useful in, identifying (often hidden) value and opportunity.

Although each of the above takes time to master, the investment in developing systems thinkers is worth the time and effort. Ultimately, health organizations practicing systems thinking will be able to step up to the next level of thinking in order to solve problems and create their desired futures. Having done so, they will have greater control over their destiny and be more nimble in responding to environmental changes.

Chapter 2: Associated Theories of Systems Thinking

Introflection

Today, healthcare delivery, and the integration of health systems at any level, too often suffers from reductionism and silo-like organizational models. General systems theory and other associated "integrative" theories can be used to clearly and concisely understand health organization structures, processes and outcomes and their interactions within a health system at all levels. Theories such as theoretical biology, chaos, complexity theory, and ecology explain how patterns of behavior drive a system's ability to adapt or not adapt in response to internal and external forces. Systems theories and integrative theories such as change, information, and communication theories can help leaders understand how healthcare and community health systems behave and provide a means to precisely assess, visualize, and analyze an organization within the system. These theories offer an understanding of the organization as a system, a necessity in the complex arena of health care and the broad scope of public health, to lead organizations effectively and efficiently to achieve organizational and community goals.

The theories that follow, while often emanating from the biological and information sciences, have been adapted for use in the social sciences. Before you proceed in reviewing these theories and consider their association to systems thinking, it may be helpful to read this passage from Hoover and Donovan's *Elements of Social Scientific Thinking.*[21]

> "After several thousand years of human history, we still have to face the fact that the process of naming things is difficult. Language emerges essentially by agreement. You and I and the other members of the family (tribe, state, nation, world) agree for example to call things that twinkle in the sky *stars*. Unfortunately, these agreements may not be precise. In common usage, the term "star" covers a multitude of objects, big and small, hot and cold, solid and gaseous.
>
> To call a thing by a precise name is the beginning of understanding, because it is the key to the procedure that allows the mind to grasp reality and its many relationships. It makes a great deal of difference whether an illness is conceived of as caused by an evil spirit or by bacteria on a binge. The concept *bacteria* is tied to a system of concepts in which there is a connection to a powerful repertory of treatments, that is, antibiotics."

General Systems Theory

General Systems Theory or the unified "science of wholeness" was initiated by biologist Ludwig von Bertanffly for two reasons: a reaction against reductionism and effort to unite the fields of science.[22,23] Reductionism, grounded in the work of Descartes and Newton, is when a system is studied by examining individual parts. Reductionism has a place in scientific or systems studies to understand how the parts work in order to understand the whole. However, most theorists in the early days of the scientific study failed to look at the system as a whole or see how all the parts are interconnected and interdependent.[24,25] According to Checkland, the aims of systems theory are to:

- *Investigate the similarities of concepts, laws, and models in various fields, and to help in useful transfers from one field to another,*
- *Encourage development of adequate theoretical models in areas which lack them,*
- *Eliminate duplication of theoretical efforts in different fields, and*
- *Promote the unity of science through improving the communication between specialists.*[24]

Today, healthcare delivery, public health, and integrated health systems are beginning to apply systems theory to facilitate sustainable changes in their organizations. For example, patient-centered medical homes (PCMH) promote unification of health care teams to enhance patient-centered care or whole teams of interdisciplinary health professionals explain treatment and family support options in oncology.

Health systems certainly are not closed systems. Being conceived by humans, who comprise them, they are open, living, and thinking, yet they are too often treated as closed and non-transparent systems. Opposing the notion of reductionism, von Bertanffly theorized systems are open to and interact with their environments.[26] For example, instead of reducing the human body to the properties of its parts, systems theory focuses on the relation between the parts, which make them a whole unit. The figure below illustrates how all systems are connected in some manner and overlap with the basic sciences. Von Bertanffly's desire to unite the different sciences is a natural evolution of this anti-reductionist theory. It was not his wish to eliminate the various fields of science (biology, chemistry, psychology, sociology, etc.), but to be able to devise a framework by which each could be analyzed and manipulated.[24]

In his article, "Systems Thinking: An Operational Perspective of the Universe," Bellinger clarified von Bertanffly's intention.

"There are fundamental structures which act across all branches of science. And, if one learns the structures, when transferring from one discipline to another, much of the learning can be transferred. When studying a new discipline, one would simply have to learn the labels on the structures in the new discipline. General Systems Theory, therefore, proposes the universe is full of systems, and each system differs from the next. There are universal laws or principles can be applied to all of them. If you learn about these universal laws, you can apply them to a specific system. A science of wholeness, General Systems Theory looks at the universe holistically rather than in parts. It is, in simplest terms, a way to understand how things work by looking for patterns responsible for behaviors and events."

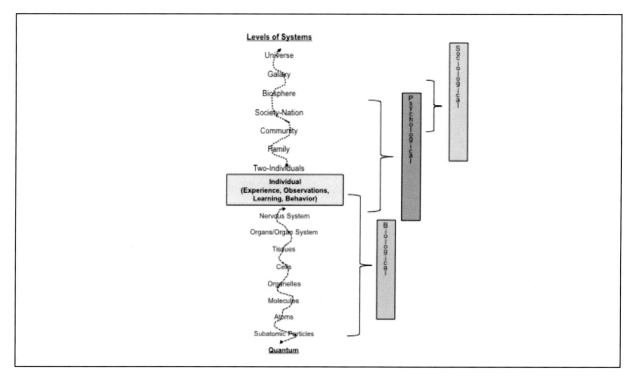

Part 1, Chapter 2, Figure 2: Modified by D. Anderson from Engel's Bio-psycho-social Model as presented in Skochelak, SE, et.al. *Health Systems Science*. Philadelphia: Elsevier. 2017

Since systems science was developed in reaction to the Newtonian view of the world, which examined things by breaking them into their parts. The discovery of subatomic particles that had qualities that could not be explained by classical physics forced scientists to look into new theories about our world.

Theoretical Biology

Systems thinking involves the whole and the parts. Theoretical Biology provides further insight into complex systems by promoting anti-reductionism and co-evolving systems.[27] Jung, Chow, and Wu found organizations require innovation in order to evolve and survive, and innovation requires ongoing leadership interactions. In other words, the system problem cannot be reduced to a single occurrence, individual or action to explain the behavior or pattern. In biology, it is nearly impossible to understand living systems by reducing them to their smallest parts.[28] Instead, living systems must be examined by looking at the interaction of their parts with each other, and their environment. Biological systems in nature are complex, in that they must interact with the environment, their ecology, and multiple other systems work to create and sustain life.[29]

Similarly, leadership decision-making impacts more than the small group of followers that have been described in traditional leadership research. Ibarra, Kilduff, and Tsai suggests network changes impact more than the work (formal system) of the organization; they also impact social identity, interactions, and relationships (informal system). The leader must be aware of the workflow, and communication changes accompany any other changes to the network.[30]

The system will attempt to evolve regardless of leader input, reward, or motivation. Theoretically, the work of leadership is part of the system and can use the position to secure resources, information, and other inputs can help shape the outcomes without predicting them.[31] When systems do not have adequate access to information, context or resources they can create mal-adaptations that can impact the organization negatively. Theoretical biology provides insights into the development of organizational context and how interconnected agents in a system relate and evolve together. The impact of inputs to the system is further explicated through the complex adaptive system concepts.[27,32,33]

Chaos and Complexity Theory

Chaos theory does not necessarily mean disordered and wild. Imagine, if external influences could be isolated, controlled, and eliminated the behaviors of systems could be predicted forever. Nothing could be further from the truth in health settings. The concepts of chaos and complexity are being applied with increasing frequency in health settings. Many experts have characterized health systems and the lack of integrated health systems as complex adaptive systems (CAS). Specifically, James Johnson states, "using, the language of systems theory, health organizations can be viewed as complex adaptive systems. Health care is complex in that it is composed of multiple, diverse, interconnected elements, and it is adaptive in that the system is capable of changing and learning from experience and its' environment."[3]

Each theory pertains to how systems behave. Many professionals believe systems behave in one of two ways: they eventually stop and stay the way they were, or they cycle between different places. Chaotic systems do not repeat themselves or stop in one place. Instead, chaotic systems are complex, unpredictable and sensitive to the conditions and changes from when they started.

Chaos refers to what might be called "ordered disorder." Chaotic systems do, in fact, follow laws can be followed and analyzed. Chaotic systems will remain unpredictable. Specific applications of chaos and complexity theory include:

- Epidemiology and infectious disease outbreak processes
- Healthcare organization mergers and consolidation
- Evidence-based healthcare practices to reduce random variation
- Biomedicine and device technology breakthroughs and uses
- Behavioral science applications to modify individual choice and lifestyles
- Sustainable development and health security at the international level
- Syndemics in applied edpidemiology

Used effectively, "chaos and complexity science" have the potential to invigorate many health settings and lead to important practical outcomes. For example, the complexity of many public health problems has led to non-linear analytic methods designed to capture the underlying dynamic processes (feedback loops, delays, cause, and effect, what if analysis) at work compared to traditional linear thinking type study designs and statistical tests. Recent interest in public health interventions has begun to see the limitations of standard methods, such as randomized trials and quasi-experiments to understand the consequences of policies and interventions designed to influence population health. Use of methods beyond simple mechanistic cause-and-effect (or risk factor–outcome) actions has stimulated interest in analytic techniques within the field of system sciences. Since systems thinking deals with complex systems complexity theory deals with assessing systems as whole units, not in pieces or parts. A complex system is functioning as whole consisting of interdependent and variable parts.

Complexity theory seeks to understand and explain dynamic systems or those capable of changing over time. Complexity theory is concerned with the predictability of underlying behavior of systems. For example, three methods used in public health proven successful in understanding complex adaptive systems: agent-based modeling, social network analysis, and system dynamics modeling. Each method has strengths and weaknesses. Each is best suited to studying some aspects of complex dynamic phenomena.

First, agent-based models involve heterogeneous actors and explore events emerging from the interaction between actors and interactions with their environments (e.g., occurrence of homelessness and increased emergency department utilization of the homeless, and prevalence of malnutrition among cohorts of the homeless).

Second, system dynamics models group actors into categories or stocks and are concerned with the flow of these conditions and factors influencing the rate at which these flows occur. This method is interested in feedback loops and unintended consequences of well-intentioned policies (i.e., occurrence of increased patient visits based on the type of insurance coverage, reimbursement methods, and incentives to produce better health in population). A fundamental concept in system dynamics is leverage points for successful interventions. These two aspects of the approach make it especially useful in policy analysis.

Finally, social network analysis can be used to understand principles of interactions between actors or examine the relationships about individuals (e.g., the spread of smoking over time within a large cohort with data associated with social media usage or organizations (e.g., exchange of resources among tobacco control agencies).

Some systems, though they are constantly changing, do so in a regular manner, while others change in a manner completely unpredictable. For example, one of the most daunting challenges is US health care reform amidst a fragmented system of health systems. The size of the system, number of stakeholders, and ever-rising costs make the problem seem almost intractable. This is especially true when national health policies swing from social to market values and incentive-based policies, chaos reigns throughout the system. To determine the patterns these policies follow it is not simple. It is the analysis of the behavior of policy decisions and these unpredictable systems chaos, and complexity theory is concerned with.

Cybernetics Theory

The study of systems theories includes the study of cybernetics. Many of the concepts applied to system science, such as communication and information, feedback, regulation, and control, are derived from cybernetics. Systems science focuses on the structure of systems. Cybernetics focuses on how systems function. Both combine structure and function as part overall systems thinking. Cybernetics focuses on the transmission of information through various communication channels. Health-care is regulation of health-conditions of patients and control of systems. Cybernetics is also the art of managing relationships.

The main area of examination in cybernetics is on the feedback loops allowing complex systems to maintain, adapt and self-organize. The internal systems of living and non-living entities work by giving commands, feeding back information on progress, and controlling by adjustment as needed, By studying the internal processes of living entities, scientists can replicate self-replicating systems in machinery or vice versa in human beings, thus creating processes and capabilities. For example, surgical robotics and remote monitoring of intensive care units is becoming more common as result of innovation and adaptation of health systems to workforce shortages and proven technologies.[22,25,34]

Cybernetics has been applied to other fields such as psychology, economics, neurophysiology, systems engineering, and the study of social systems. Medical Cybernetics investigates inter-causal networks in human biology, medical decision making and information processing structures in the living organism. For example, according to many studies, nearly 70% of US adults are either overweight or obese, diabetes rates have increased 27 percent the last five years, and at least 250,000 thousand people die of a heart attack each year. Many experts think health problems can be mitigated by regulating someone's lifestyle. The study of cybernetics within a group or with a friend may help people to adopt a healthy way of life. Thus, cybernetic theories contribute to understanding and developing greater individual self-determination, and greater understanding, tolerance, and a variety of responses to situations and people leading to helping people to interact and respond effectively to urges and situations do not contribute to better health.

Social Network Theory

Social network theory is the study of how people, organizations or groups interact with others inside their network or across organizational boundaries. Understanding the theory involves examining individual pieces starting with the largest element: networks, and working down to the smallest element: actors. As systems thinkers, studying relationships and methods of interaction is critical to sustainable change. For example understanding stakeholder's interests, capacities, and constraints are crucial when developing sustainable initiatives such as smoke-free city blocks, more walking and cycling paths, or speeding cameras. Social networks are seen as important in the process by which health professionals adopt (or fail to adopt) innovations in their respective environments.

Social networks are synonymous with communities: comprised of actors and relationships between actors. These actors or nodes can be individuals, organizations, or health policy decision makers. The ministry of health (MOH) in a small country can be viewed as a social network, while non-governmental organizations can represent nodes inside the network or MOH. Social scientists explore ego-centric, socio-centric, and open-system networks. Ego-centric networks are connected to a single node or individual. For example, healthcare administrators are linked with peers. Socio-centric networks are closed networks by default. Two examples are patients in a waiting room or nurses in the intensive care unit. In open-system networks, boundaries lines are vague. Examples may be connections between various health systems, chains of influencers of a particular issue such as pharmaceutical price regulation.

Social networks provide a powerful approach to health behavior change. Social network interventions have been successfully utilized for a range of health behaviors including HIV risk practices, smoking, exercise, dieting, family planning, bullying, and mental health. The relationship between health behaviors and social network attributes demonstrate the potential for improving the health of a population by applying social norms, modeling, and social rewards and factors of social identity and social rewards to sustain healthier community interventions. Use of a combination of mobile and telehealth and face-to-face networks for promoting health behavior change could result in community breakthroughs. Social scientists and health leaders should be concerned with the interactions between various nodes of a network. These connections or relationships help us understand and to find breakthrough points for change.

Information and Communication Theory

Information and communication theory studies the transmission, reception, and processing of information. More specifically, communication theory looks at the measurement of information with numbers, in what language or code the information is presented, and the ability of the communication system to send, receive, and decode the information back to its original language. Information theory is concerned with the adaptability of a message through a particular channel for maximum transmission. In health informatics, information theory can be a benefit by improving structure — the capacity of facilities and capabilities and qualification of the personnel and organization, process — changes in volume, cost and appropriateness of activities, outcome — change in health care status attributed to an object being evaluated. The major challenges, however, would be initial implementation and acceptance. At the same time, communication alone will not solve all problems. For example, electronic medical appointment reminders may not be helpful without transportation, food, and housing support for certain populations.

Communication should be targeted at improving health. For example, health communication is the practice of communicating promotional health information, such as in public health campaigns, health education, and between health professionals and patients. Asynchronous communication also has the potential to significantly improve the quality of care. The easy access to the Internet should enable continuous inquiries and feedback between patients and the health care system actors. The internet has already changed patients' ability to self-manage aspects of their care. One of the fastest growing uses of the Internet is as a source of medical information from third parties making patients more informed and, unfortunately, sometimes misinformed.[35] The purpose is to influence health choices by improving health literacy. Health communication strategies must be tailored for audiences and the situation to enhance health or avoid specific health risks. Health communication may be employed to:

- Increase knowledge and awareness of a population's health issue
- Influence behaviors towards adopting a healthy lifestyle
- Demonstrate healthy practices and patterns or habits
- Demonstrate benefits of behavior changes in health outcomes
- Advocate a position on a health reform or policy
- Increase demand or support for health services
- Argue against misconceptions about health
- Advance health literacy and empowerment
- Mobilize communities before and during a health crisis

Communication is a series of multi-dimensional transactions influenced by many factors. In health promotion, the successful exchange of information between practitioners and affected populations should be planned and implemented.

Change Management Theory

In today's changing health environment, technological advancements and medical devices such as "apps" can challenge health professionals in many ways. Implementing a change in practice typically produces anxiety or fear of failure leading to resistance. Change management theories such as Lewin's and Lippitt's theory can lead to a better understanding of how change affects the organizational systems, identify barriers for successful implementation. Change management theories are useful for identifying opposing forces impacting human behavior during the change, therefore overcoming resistance and leading to acceptance. Planned change in practice is necessary for a wide range of reasons, but it can be challenging to implement. Medication errors in hospital settings lead to consequences for health teams and patients. Errors can be reduced significantly through the use of technology improves patient care and saves time for busy nurses. Bar-coded medication administration use scanning devices to compare bar codes on identification bands with coded medications, and verifies the medications against the record, thereby reducing medication errors. However, perceptions and misperceptions may prevail during implementation. Understanding and using change management theories help leaders increase the likelihood of success.

Reflection

Both humans and organizations are complex systems. Systems theories provide a framework to understand and solve complicated health problems and system issues within and outside a health organization. Systems thinking should drive health, leaders, and policy makers to look at the smaller interdependent components of the system, within the larger system. Without looking at the larger system as a whole, the system could be compromised. The interdependency of the components means changes to any subsystem could result in a domino effect, thus changing the system as a whole. Systems theories are helpful in understanding organic systems, or systems involving living beings. As organic systems are always interacting with each other and with their environment, the system is always changing. Leaders can understand how humans and organizations interact with each other, their environment, and the intricacies of systems. In health organizations where we have people, processes, and structures, there are multiple systems and sub-systems involved. Each of the systems are inter-related. Leaders and health professionals need to be systems thinkers in order to facilitate sustainable change in organizations and communities, while guarding against unintended consequences. When complex systems, such as whole communities or countries have the capacity to adapt to its changing environment, it is considered a complex adaptive system. These systems, including the social determinants of health, beliefs, and culture, are also a part of a larger global system influencing humans, organizations, and policy.

Chapter 3: The Health System as a "System of Systems"

Introflection

An all too common challenge in systems thinking is understanding the whole "system" or big picture. As a quick reminder of an earlier discussion in this book, a system is a set of two or more elements where the 1) behaviors of each element affects the behavior of the whole system, 2) behaviors of the elements and their effects, on the whole, are interdependent, and 3) elements of a system are connected independent subgroups and cannot be separated. For example, a system comprises interactions (feedback loops, flows, and stocks) such as an ICU Nurse's interactions with the medical, surgical unit, materials management or discharge functions or subsystems. However, the ICU is part of a much larger health system or system of systems.

Systems Components

Systems can be comprised of hardware, software, wetware (the brain) technology, human behavior, or as is most common, a combination. The "system" can take the form of a problem such as preventing harm or preadmission penalties. This issue has an external context such as payment policies or families as caregivers and structure such as the process by which patients move through the systems to alternative settings. In fact, preventing harm or preventing readmissions extends beyond a typical hospital's walls. These problems and subsequent opportunities should challenge leaders to systematically rethink their current value proposition such as the relentless pursuit of zero harm throughout the continuum of care before admission, during the care process, discharge to a home or health setting, and patient/ family engagement.

As stated previously, a system is a group of interacting, interrelated, or interdependent components to form a complex unified whole. All systems contain inputs: raw material, energy, and resources processed to produce outputs. Examples include information, funding, health team's effort, provider's time, and individual effort. Elements or components are things, parts, or substances to make up the system. These parts may be humans, material, equipment, etc. Elements have measurable or descriptive characteristics such as color, size, volume, quantity, temperature, and mass. Throughput is the processes used by a system to convert materials, intellect, or energy into products or services usable by either the system itself or the environment. Examples include thinking, physical examination of patients, diagnosing, planning, decision-making, writing prescriptions, taking vital signs, operating on a patient, constructing, etc. The output is the result from the system's throughput or processing of technical, social, financial & cerebral. Examples include health services, better health, software programs, documents, and decisions, etc. The figure below provides a conceptual perspective of the health system and the typical input, process, and output approach.

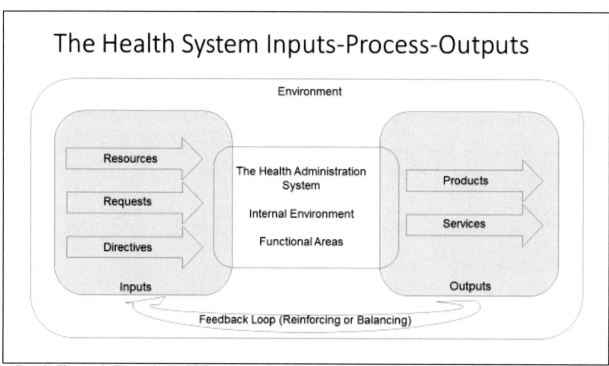

Part 1, Chapter 3, Figure 3: Health System as a Set of Inputs-Processes-Outputs. Adapted by D. Anderson from Denhardt RB, et.al. *Managing Human Behavior in Public and Nonprofit Organizations* 3rd ed. Los Angeles: Sage. 2013

Also, a system's components can be physical objects such as the various parts that make up an intensive care unit (ICU) or medical group practice. These components can be intangible: culture, processes; relationships; policies; information; interpersonal interactions; and internal states of mind such as feelings, values, and beliefs. The keys for systems thinking are mutual interaction, which implies something occurs between the parts to maintain the existence or performance of the system. The parts are, therefore, interdependent and interconnected. The loss or breakdown of any one part will affect the function of the whole.[36] Feedback in systems is critical. Feedback is information about some indicator of data, patient flow, or energy processing used to evaluate and monitor the system and guide it to effective performance. How many patients were seen in a 2-hour clinic? How many medical errors were committed in a hospital? Why were mistakes made? Hospital accreditation reports are examples as are patient satisfaction surveys, sales reports, and test results.

Systems thinking challenges leaders to apply a process of systemic inquiry to uncover assumptions, biases, see the connections between systems and subsystems inside and outside the walls of their institution. For example, preventable patient harm is often associated with human error. Such errors are often met with blame and punishment. The "system" in systems thinking is a flexible construct to help in understanding complexity, relations, and generating creative solutions. Systems thinking should drive a culture of continuous process improvement thus providing a much less threatening context than "name, blame, and shame" approaches to improving organizations or communities. The analysis and understanding of the aspects of systems, and how issues are related, is critical to systems thinking and leadership. Without a clear perspective on the system itself, systems thinking will fail.

Subsystems and Dynamic Systems

A subsystem is a smaller system within a larger system. Subsystems can operate in parallel or entangled with each other. Information systems are subsystems. The medical staff as an organization is a subsystem of the hospital. Health care systems are categorized based on the level of care provided within each subsystem: acute care, extended care, home care, and ambulatory care. Also, preventive and self-care could be regarded as a subsystem.

A dynamic system continuously influences and changes its environment and is being influenced and modified by its environment. Dynamic systems are usually composed of components structured and interrelated in such a way a change in one component affects other components or elements of the larger system. A hospital in any country or district, i.e. the Cayo District of Belize is an example of a system where it influences its environment (health, quality of life) and is affected by the environment such as policies and local needs. Evidence-based practice in health care is an example of how health care services attempt to address the dynamics of healthcare delivery and decision to reduce variation in care or allow processes in systems to become stable, so that a team can customize care or adapt to the dynamics of the system.

Types of Systems and Subsystems

The types of systems can range from simple (filling a glass of water) to incredibly complex (climate change). They are always working to maintain a level of stability in a dynamic environment. They do so by creating feedback loops using inputs and outputs. Inputs influence system behaviors over time. For example, an open system interacts with its environment exchanging raw materials and energy for services and goods produced by the system. Health facilities, hospitals, nursing homes, families, humans, and other care systems are examples of open systems. Hospitals deliver healing services through practice, health professionals, training, and knowledge. In return, it receives money, raw materials, appreciation, and energy from its environment. Systems typically have goals. The goal is the purpose for existence. Examples include treating patients, educating student nurses, and so on. Many variations of system types exist. Understanding the basics of system types is helpful:

1. *Closed Systems*: Closed systems do not need to interact with the environment. Nothing enters or leaves it. Closed systems are entirely self-contained, not influenced by external events, and eventually die. Closed health systems are closed off from the environment. Interaction and knowledge are transmitted within the closed system. Closed systems can starve themselves with a lack of outside information since the flow of information stays within the system. It has no chance to interact with or build on knowledge from the outer environment

2. *Natural Systems*: A living being's body and health systems have enormous numbers and complex of components and interactions among their components.

3. *Designed Systems*: Although treadmills can be complex, it is not intricately linked to a system unless it becomes part of a physical therapy department, a section in the clinical pathway, or feature in the marketing brochure on health and wellness. If the treadmill

breaks down, the impact can be felt throughout the human made but a non-living system. Thus human-made nonliving systems become interdependent and are more open with their connections.

4. *Open Systems*: Open systems interact with its environment to exist. For example, people rely on external conditions to survive. These conditions are why addressing social determinants of health is imperative. They need shelter, to take in air, food, and water, and in return, they leave waste. How well communities address these basic needs drives the ability of a population to thrive. A system interacts with its environment, by receiving inputs from and delivering outputs to the outside, is called an open system. They possess permeable boundaries, permit interaction across organizational boundaries where new information and ideas are readily absorbed thus allowing the incorporation of improved processes. They can adapt more quickly to changes in the external environment in which they operate. For example, health professionals learn the value of changing microsystems within their control; people, machines, data to direct patient care while public health professionals concentrate on prevention of disease and population health management. However, these microsystems are subsystems within a macro system; hospitals, nursing homes, clinics, and public health departments. Today's challenges urge leadership to integrate all microsystems such as public health, occupational safety, social services, and community outreach agencies as a means to build healthier communities.

5. *Continuous Learning Systems*: Most results in the world today are derived from interactions within systems composed of machines, computers, and people. The "thinking" in continuous learning systems is an ability to create new ideas, innovate, make improvements never seen before, and sometimes to act purposefully without regard for survival. A continuous learning system is a complex system populated by humans who interact with each other. Humans may have diverse and contradictory purposes, but they are always learning. A continuous learning system has goals separate from survival and a capability to innovate purposefully. Lifelong learning systems always learn and structure their learning. As robotics and artificial intelligence (AI) continues to infuse our lives, we will see more of these kinds of systems. Human thinking will soon, and already has in many ways, be augmented by AI, not simply for efficiency but also for enhanced creativity. Many futurists now comfortably discuss "transhumanism." With the use of Watson and hospital based robots, we are basically at the threshold of the vast potential this has for human health – both in health delivery and public health.

Health Systems as Open and Continuous Learning Systems of Systems

As the environment influences the system, the system also influences the environment. Allowing a system to be open ultimately sustains growth and serves its parent environment, and so both have a stronger probability of survival. Continuous learning systems have a second unique characteristic: creative ability to use what is known and go beyond the level of expectations and create disruptive innovations or breakthrough process.[37] Systems thinking in the context of openness is an approach designed to embrace the dynamics of changing health reform landscape, global public health challenges, and prevent unintended consequences. Systems thinking can mitigate many dysfunctions in health organizations by re-perceiving themselves as open and thinking systems within a larger system. Many have become well organized and recognize their success is outside the boundaries of their organization and individual thinking. Integrated health systems are not an abstraction but a current and future reality.

Several health organizations engage in community partnerships, have system-wide information systems and teams of clinicians and health system integrators to provide care efficiently, reliably, and safely. Some have characterized these organizations as fully "integrated" delivery systems that own the hospitals, employ physicians, use a single information system, and play the role of health insurance plan. Examples include the Veterans Health Administration, Kaiser Permanente, Intermountain Healthcare, Cleveland Clinics, and Geisinger Health System. A closer look at these systems reveals they are open, thinking, and learning health systems. Through thinking and learning, systems intentionally improve and respond to opportunities in the environment as part of the larger system of systems.

Reflection

Unlike closed systems, open systems, especially health systems exchange feedback with the external environment and other systems. Open systems are systems, for which their inputs, processes, outputs, goals, assessment and evaluation, and external relations, and continuous learning are necessary. These systems also extend into the communities they serve and beyond into larger national and perhaps even global systems. Open systems include permeable boundaries, monitor external environments for opportunities, and continuously exchange feedback with other systems. Successful health systems are open, transparent, and continuously learning at all levels. Michael Friesen and James Johnson, in their book *The Success Paradigm* describe this kind of health organization as embracing the seminal work of Peter Senge, known as the "Fifth Discipline" in which the successful and sustainable organizations readily embrace systems thinking, personal mastery, creative mental models, shared vision, and team learning. Friesen and Johnson's success paradigm will be discussed more in Part II.

Chapter 4: Levels of Integration in Complex Adaptive Health Systems

Introflection

In the previous chapters, the basics, foundations, and types of systems were introduced. Systems thinking tends to embrace democratic principles of organization in which all voices have meaning and are sought, and authority is distributed. Systems have an internal process where there are continued exchanges between subsets of the system. To make effective change in any portion of a complex dynamic health system, interactions and interfaces of its parts need to be understood. As such, addressing the health system at any level along with understanding the degree of integration in the context of complex adaptive health systems is imperative.

In complex systems, organization behaviors appear to emerge somewhat spontaneously. They are referred to as emergent behaviors or self-organized patterns of behaviors. An example of emergent, self-organized behaviors exists in biological systems such as flocking birds and schools of fishes. Another example is how the brain self-organizes into neuronal networks of emergent behavior patterns such as walking, sleeping, or heart rates.

The US system of agriculture is a case in point where a system can transform without a master plan. In the 20th century, agriculture transformed from a disorganized, costly, and inefficient enterprise to a productive and cost-effective system. Farming improvements were attributable to continuous experimentation, measurement, and learning. A similar opportunity exists with health systems.[38] However, in the transformation of agriculture there have been many unintended consequences, damage to the environment, impact on small farms, and the rise of agro-business, with food companies having dominance over farming. Fortunately, as the reader will see in this chapter complex adaptive systems, such as health care, agriculture, transportation, and education will change as needed to continue to survive and as we see it, with the help of systems thinking, actually thrive.

Health Systems as Complex Adaptive Systems

Many leaders think decomposing overall system performance into component elements such as quality, cost, and access will drive better design. However, this approach tends to separate and isolate analyses only to formulate isolated recommendations with trade-offs. This method works for developing cell phones and retail systems. However, healthcare and the promotion of healthier communities is considerably more complicated. As you now know, a system is greater than the sum of its parts and requires assessment of the whole system rather than individual parts of the system – why are so many homeless people presenting at the emergency room? Second, though each sub-system is a self-contained unit, it is part of a wider entity – what are the goals and interests of the local community health system or helping agencies? Third, every system is an information system and must be analyzed regarding how suitable information is transmitted between units – are we sharing the right information with the right actors and stakeholders and vice versa? Fourth, open and continuous learning health systems mean high interaction with and between the system and environment – understanding the social determinants of health and communicating the impacts. And finally, the purposes of the sub-systems must be aligned with the purpose of the system as a whole – do all actors and stakeholders understand the elements of the Triple Aim: Improve population health, increase the experience of care, and reduce the cost per capita and social determinants of health? Are there common areas where partnerships can be formed to address mutual goals? Upon exploring these and myriad other questions, health leaders, social scientists, and policy-makers must think and sometime, re-think regarding health system levels and interfaces.

Complex adaptive health systems at any level or context are typically nonlinear and dynamic or in perpetual motion. A health leader may view patterns and behaviors as random or chaotic, yet rarely seek out the types of interactions between systems much less their own. Complex adaptive systems are composed of independent agents whose behaviors are based on goals, interests, processes, policies, and culture or social rules rather than system dynamics. As such, goals and actions are likely to conflict and agents tend to adapt to each other's behaviors. Agents, in turn, experiment and gain experience, and change their behaviors accordingly. Thus overall system transforms over time. Adaptation and learning result in self-organization. Behavior patterns emerge instead of purposeful design. These emergent behaviors range from valuable innovations, partisanship, to accidents given no single touch points exist in the system. System behaviors become unpredictable and unstable. Consequently, behaviors of complex adaptive health systems should be easily influenced rather than controlled.

As described by Anderson and Johnson, complex systems behave differently than more simple systems, and thus provide special challenges for systems thinkers and leaders. In fact critical thinking should go beyond what is beyond a simple event and providing a seemingly simple solution. The figure below challenges leaders to look beyond the event. Critical and systems thinking is required to look for patterns and hidden formal and informal structures. Rather than focus on the event, the causes and effects throughout the larger system must be considered. The goal is to uncover systemic patterns or trends and structures to understand how to develop sustainable solutions rather than fixes that eventually fail. Digging into the structures of vicious cycles of reoccurring problems can be reversed. Only by thinking critically, can health leaders identify higher level, creative, and innovative long term interventions or policies.

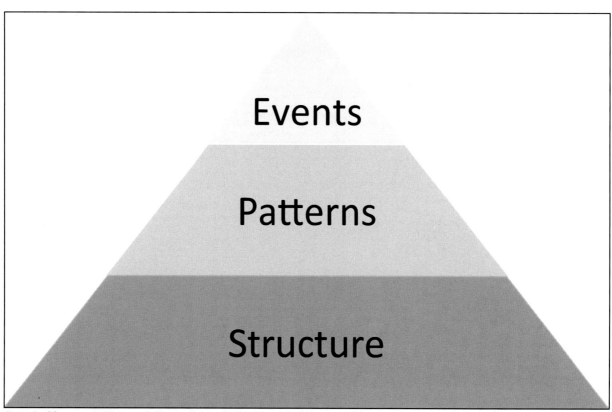

Part 1, Chapter 4, Figure 4: Basic Critical Thinking Model adopted by J. Johnson and D. Anderson from Anderson, V. and Johnson, L. Systems Thinking Basics. Acton, MA: Pegasus. 1997

The authors assert, "In action, a complex system appears to have many variables, many factors at play, and many semi-independent but interlocking components."[39] Further defining characteristics of complex systems include the following:

1. *Complex systems tend to be self-stabilizing.* The causal loop diagram below illustrates how a systems is likely to contain many balancing feedback loops, each of which serves to keep some smaller component or subsystem in balance with the larger more complex system. An example would be the various units of the National Institutes of Health remaining on the cutting edge of research within their domain while also serving the larger purpose and mission of medical research.
2. *Complex systems are purposeful.* Despite all the feedback loops and balancing loops, these systems often seem to function with a mind of their own. An example of this is the experience of a hospital CEO who can't grasp the cause of high nursing staff turnover in their organization.
3. *Complex systems are capable of using feedback to modify their behavior.* All systems do this, providing an essential opportunity for change and growth – i.e. adaptation and innovation. An example would be a health organization forming a partnership with the local Council on Aging and then organizing and integrated approach to elder care.
4. *Complex systems can modify their environments.* Since systems seek to fulfill a purpose they can modify their behavior accordingly. Often in doing so they also alter their environments. Essential to changing any environment is the need to identify the links

between the system and its environment. An example would be using systems thinking to address water quality issues in a community such as Flint, Michigan.
5. *Complex systems are capable of replicating, maintaining, repairing, and organizing themselves.* This is sometimes referred to as reinvention or organizational transformation. A healthcare example would be the incredible growth in scope and scale of the Cleveland Clinics over the past decade.

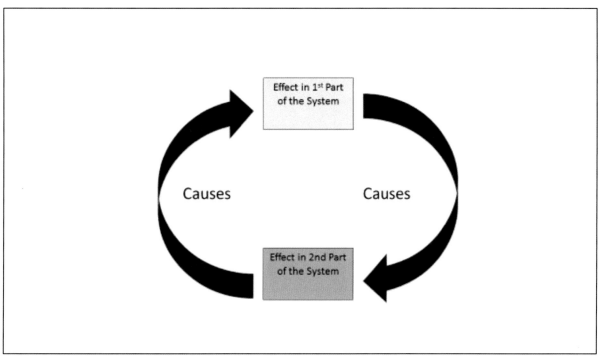

Part 1, Chapter 4, Figure 5: Simple Causal Feedback Loop Diagram; Created by D. Anderson

Effective health systems design must consider and assume complexity at each level. Viewing the overall health care delivery as a system of systems or networks at any level is a start. As much as possible, complex health systems should be designed. Design should begin with the recognition of the health enterprise—as a system with levels and interactions—healthcare, public health, and non-health stakeholder organizations. The strategy should focus on each level of complexity where it can be leveraged or influenced. The World Health Organization (WHO) strongly embraces this empowering perspective by promulgating a framework of health systems building blocks. As described by James Johnson in the book, *Comparative Health Systems*, where he and colleagues studied 20 different health systems around the world, "Even though every health system is unique in its given social and cultural environment, it has common elements that are necessary to function. These building blocks not only help us to understand health systems better but also provide opportunities for system improvement."[15] Friesen and Johnson in *The Success Paradigm,* describe these building blocks as "critical success factors" that are essential to a health system's survival and sustainability.[40]

Table 1
Health Systems Building Blocks (Critical Success Factors)

Service Delivery	Medical Technology
Good health services are those that deliver effective, safe, quality personal and non-personal health interventions to those who need them, when and where needed, with minimum waste of resources.	A well-functioning health system ensures equitable access to essential medical products, drugs, vaccines, and technologies of assured quality, safety, efficacy, and cost-effectiveness, and their scientifically sound and cost-effective use.
Health Workforce	**Health Financing**
A well-performing health workforce is one that works in ways that are responsive, fair, and efficient to achieve the best health outcomes possible, given available resources and circumstances (i.e., there are sufficient staff, fairly distributed; they are competent, responsive, and productive).	A good health financing system raises adequate funds for health, in ways that ensure people can use needed services and are protected from financial catastrophe or impoverishment associated with having to pay for them. It provides incentives for providers and users to be efficient.
Health Information	**Leadership and Governance**
A well-functioning health information system is one that ensures the production, analysis, dissemination, and use of reliable and timely information on health determinants, health system performance, and health status.	Leadership and governance involves ensuring that strategic policy frameworks exist and are combined with effective oversight, coalition building, regulation, attention to system design, and accountability.

Author created from WHO framework. *Systems Thinking for Health Systems Thinking*. Geneva: WHO Press. 2009

The challenge then is to think of the system in larger parts to include those outside the system such as the social determinants of health in the public health system or other systems, which present opportunities for collaboration and partnership. For example, thinking about systems in levels and interfaces is important in global health especially international development. The figure below illustrates the power of systems thinking using causal loop diagrams or CLDs.

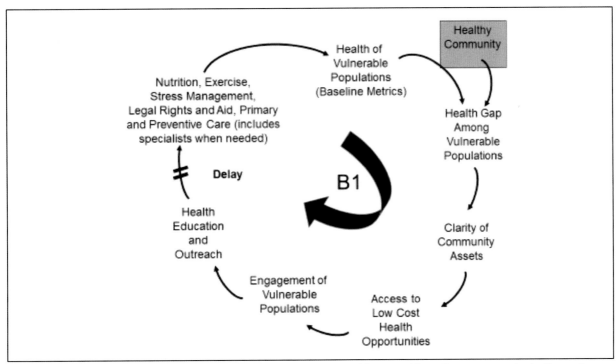

Part 1, Chapter 4, Figure 6: Example of Feedback Loop Using Building Healthier Communities As An Example. Adapted by D. Anderson from Stroh D. Systems Thinking For Social Change: A Practical Guide to Solving Complex Problems, Avoiding Unintended Consequences, and Achieving Lasting Results

One of the great observations is the need for the global health sector to renew its focus on health systems strengthening to create stable economies and minimize risk to traveling diseases. Experts acknowledge the success of disease-specific approaches in recent years, yet point out how enabling environments or the social determinants of health and system-level interventions hold more promise for improving health outcomes in communities.[41] However, several distinctions must be made to broaden the health leader's horizons about healthcare to a system of producing health. Understanding the levels and interfaces will enhance the health leader's ability to generate sustainable systems.[19]

Health Systems Levels and Integration (Or Lack Of)

Health systems are fragile and must be viewed regarding levels and interfaces. Systems theories inform leaders about the nature and behaviors of systems. This fragility implies the interdependent nature of health systems at an individual, organizational, community, national, and global level. For example, at the lowest level, patients such as an elderly person who has fallen and broken their hip move between different levels of health care such. While in the acute care setting many processes and subsystems are at work: admission, surgery, administration of pain medication, and physical care including physical therapy. The patient can get out of bed, walk using a walker, and begin eating well.

Systems are multidimensional structures capable of interaction with other systems on planning and sharing resources. Systems-based planning must be interactive. For example, the elderly patient who broke their hip is transferred to extended care. They are not critically ill but requires round the clock assistance. When the patient can move safely around and no longer needs 24-hour care, they can be transferred home. This action requires coordination of care beyond the acute care setting and presents additional risks to safety and readmission. Therefore, ends have to be clear before means are discussed between actors and stakeholders in the system. For example, in the case of the elderly patient, a Home Health Care nurse verifies patient safety and transition into the home environment. A plan for home PT is established, and care continues at home until the patient is independent. Going beyond the care scenario, the systems approach would also consider the community-based opportunities for recreation and physical activity, social support, and education about safety and self-care. Perhaps the home itself needs to be re-engineered in some way or a dietician enlisted to assure healthy eating habits for bone health and muscle development. One can even envision further to consider health policy around Medicare and Medicaid to help assure follow-up care.

Systems thinking concepts can and must be extended to health care settings. To improve health care operations, understanding the system's influence can drive improvements. Clinical care is embedded in an interconnected system, however, from a policy perspective, accountable care organizations (ACO) and payment reform (i.e., bundled payment) are challenging health systems to think beyond direct clinical attention and focus on coordination of care. Systems-based planning must have feedback systems to make the interdependencies visible and manageable. In this case, measures of the experience of care, resources consumed, and patient safety are considered feedback loops. While this illustration focused on one level of care the interfaces between systems become necessary. This case also illustrates how complexity sets in when other levels and interfaces intervene. For example, the ability to pay, the source of payment, the capacity of local health services, need for other types of health or community health professionals, alternative therapies, and lifestyle or behavior changes are needed.

These levels and interfaces can be divided into the following:

1. Individual
2. Team
3. Organization
4. System
5. National
6. Global

Systems at any level have the ability to learn to adapt to changing components and environment. For example, community organizations are bound by social networks, norms, standards, and other invisible factors thus affecting relationships at the individual and team levels. Complex-adaptive health systems are made up of interacting components at each level whose interactions may be complex and nonlinear and whose components are diverse and have a capacity for learning. Institutions or organizations within the community may follow the rules, regulations, policies and create simple or informal structures according to the influences of community and national levels. Health leaders can either by reactive or proactive in their approaches to creating sustainable solutions.

Individual

This level pertains to an individual's needs, knowledge, attitudes, and beliefs. It also pertains to an individual's physical and behavioral health, wellness, and resilience. As a patient needs, preferences, and demographics define factors associated with a patient-centered health care system. Today, the availability or non-availability of information and measures drives increasing expectations for changes in the system to improve quality, efficiency, and effectiveness. Overall, the role of the patient as a passive recipient of care has increasingly transformed to that of a more active participant.

The fragmented health system, combined with the burden of chronic disease and the need for continuous care, has forced patients to be more active in the design, coordination, and implementation of their recovery process. Considering the transformed roles and needs of patients, their interdependencies with other actors at other levels in the health system have expanded and become more complex. At the same time, opportunities exist to improve the performance of a fragmented and dysfunctional healthcare delivery system.

Further, patient-centeredness is challenging health professionals to consider patients and their families as part of the coordination of care process. The level of responsibility patients and family members assume will differ depending on the patient and type of health issues. Some prefer to delegate while others want to be full partners in decision making. In either case, however, patients need a free exchange of information and communication with their healthcare teams as well as with the organizations providing support to the healthcare teams. For example, both patients and healthcare teams need to be able to communicate needs and preferences as part of the coordination of care process. Access to the same information streams is critical.

Team

The health care team, the second level of the health system, consists of a group of care providers, family members, and others. Their efforts result in the delivery of care to a patient or population of patients. The health care team is the core building block of a "micro-system." This system is defined as the smallest unit within an organization [or across multiple organizations]. It is replicable--contains the necessary human, financial, and technological resources to do its work.[42] It could also include public health and community support agencies impacting the social determinants of health related to the patient's healing process.

A health team microsystem includes a defined patient population and an information environment to support health professionals, caregivers, patients including support staff, equipment, and facilities.[43] Ideally, the role of the microsystem is to standardize care processes with current evidence, stratify patients based on need and provide the best evidence-based care within each stratum. Customization of care to meet individual needs for patients with complex health problems must follow.[44]

The role and needs of health care teams have undergone changes similar to their patients. For example, the increases in medical knowledge, the proliferation of specialties, and burden of providing chronic care requires more interaction and interdependence across organizations or institutional settings. The slow adaptation from individual clinicians to team-based health care has been influenced by the lack of formal training in teamwork, a culture of autonomy, and the absence of an information infrastructure, and incentives to facilitate change.

At present, few care teams or clinical microsystems are considered the primary agents of patient-centered care. Unwarranted variations in care are common, even for conditions and patient populations where evidence-based or best practice protocols are standard [45]. Even though many clinicians accept the value of "evidence-based medicine" and recognize they cannot deliver evidence-based care on their own, many barriers exist to changing practices. All of these prevent systems thinking to care delivery. Thus, tailoring evidence-based care to meet individual patient's needs remains an elusive goal.

For care teams to be patient-centered, processes and rules should be transformed into being more responsive to the needs of patients, involve them and their families earlier, and provide personalized care. Teams must provide patients with continuous, convenient, and timely access to quality care. This approach, a systems approach must include ensuring effective communication and coordination between the patient and other members of the care team is constant.[35]

Organization

The next level of the health system is the organization (e.g., hospital, clinic, nursing home, public health department) provides infrastructure and complementary resources to support the healthcare teams. The organization is a critical lever of change in the health system. It provides an overall climate and culture for change through decision-making systems, operating systems, and human resource practices.[44] The organization provides decision-making systems, information systems, operating systems, and processes (financial, administrative, human resource, and clinical) to coordinate care through the experience of care to support teams of teams. Allocation and flow of human, material, and financial resources and information in support of care teams must be optimized. Typically, this includes a hospital, clinic, nursing home, etc. that supports the work of care teams by providing infra- structure and complementary resources. The organizational infrastructure also influences effective delivery of care to the patient or citizens in the community and social support services. Ensuring health professionals have the correct tools and skills is an essential element of infrastructure. For example, the electronic health record is one of the most significant advances for the healthcare team, patients, and the organizations. Another component of the organization is leadership. Without leadership, progress or transformation will not occur.

Organizations (systems) have inputs, processes, and outputs. Inputs include resources such as personnel, equipment, computers, raw materials, money, technologies, and information. Inputs are processed to produce the outputs. Outputs are the results of the processes in an organization. Outputs can be goods or services. Organizations produce services such as providing health care, protecting against diseases and providing nutritional services. Feedback comes from multiple sources: managers, workers, patients, media, and community leaders. Organizations are composed of subsystems. The number of subsystems determines the complexity of an organization. Each subsystem has boundaries, inputs, processes and outputs. Examples are departments, units, projects, teams, or processes. Organizations are defined by their mission, plans, goals, policies and procedures, and organizational charts. Feedback within the organizational system is maintained or controlled by policies, processes, and procedures, budgets and quality management programs. Health organizations face many challenges. In response to the escalating costs, government and third-party payers have shifted a growing share of the costs to providers and patients.

Social groups and networks exist and interact to produce, consume and exchange goods, services, and ideas. Understanding health professions socialization is helpful for understanding organizations as systems. Continuous feedback between the different components of the system ensures the system is accomplishing the goals of the organization (system). A system can be the entire organization, or any of its departments, groups, or processes.

System

Organizational systems are more complex than some other systems, in part due to their interactive infrastructure. There are two distinct sections of an organizational system, the internal and the external system. The internal system consists of a variety of parts, including the products or services produced, personnel, the materials and tools used to create products or services. The external system is everything outside the organization: Competitors, economy, financial conditions, environment, regulations, politics, and the community. Both the internal and external systems are not only interacting within themselves but are also interacting with each other. Understanding these interactions and finding opportunities to leverage improvements is the crux of systems thinking.

There are hundreds of other people and dozens of institutions working to make interaction possible. They constitute the healthcare system. For example, the six system building-blocks, previously discussed, to achieve health system goals: service delivery, health workforce, information systems, access to medicines, financing, and leadership or governance.[19] These elements set the stage for sustainable development. Each of these elements provides opportunities to improve healthcare delivery or prevent disease outbreaks. Beyond the medical research and development to produce new vaccines or treatments, sustainable development includes innovations in areas like supply chain systems to reduce clinic stock-outs in countries such as Senegal or financing such as out outpatient smart cards in Kenya.[46] How we assess system-level improvements is still a challenge: we need better measurement of these system elements to target the optimal leverage points, and the best interventions for a given system will remain highly context-dependent and difficult to design.

There's a further level of complexity that gets surfaced through systems thinking. This level requires us to go beyond merely seeing the impact of system elements on healthcare, and also see the complex impacts system elements have on other system elements. These subsystems get more complex and interconnected. Systems thinking is highly concerned with flows/stocks, feedback loops, sustainability, resilience, and hierarchy of the organization. At the system level, health leaders and policy-makers must keep in mind the key lessons of systems thinking: elements interact in unexpected and counterintuitive ways. For example, the policies affecting the availability of health professionals goes through several channels: compensation, law, regulations, and immigration.

Similarly, access to care depends on the transportation infrastructures and social networks. These can be improved with capital investments (e.g. roads, new health facilities), financing, and information systems (i.e. cell towers and telemedicine). Adjustments play out on different timelines, complicating assessments. The interactions may be unique while other elements might e relevant in some contexts, including cultural and linguistic diversity, financing, politics, or literacy. Application of systems thinking has the potential to uncover more opportunities than a linear mindset. It requires the competency to make sense of complexity at any level. This competency requires a deeper understanding of the systems and the actors or stakeholders associated with it.[16]

There's another dimension for health leaders and systems thinkers from all domains to consider, that is the shift of mindset to thinking about health, not just healthcare. The healthcare delivery system is only one element of a larger system of influencing the health of an individual or community. Social determinants of health — water and sanitation, environmental conditions, food, security, and more — have incredibly significant influence over health outcomes. These systems often provide greater opportunities to improve health, as they are often the source of negative health outcomes.[19]

National

The National level addresses the political and economic environment (e.g., regulatory, financial, payment regimes, and markets), conditions under which organizations, care teams, individual patients, and individual care providers operate.[35] The environment influences the delivery of care. Environmental factors include competition, regulation, payment systems, and demographics. Significant improvements in health and health care can be achieved when leaders base their strategy on health and health care initiatives using systems thinking.

This level influences the structure and performance of the health systems and organizations directly and indirectly. Many actors influence the health policy and reform process. The federal government influences care through reimbursement practices, regulation of private-payer and provider partnerships, and support for research and development and use of selected diagnostic and therapeutic interventions (e.g., drugs, devices, equipment, and procedures). State governments play a major role in the administration of Medicaid, as well as the education and licensure of health professionals. Private-sector purchasers of health care, are important environment-level actors influencing reimbursement of services not covered by the federal government.[35]

Federal regulations influence the nature of competition among providers and insurers. They also affect the transparency of the health care system by setting requirements related to patient safety. By exercising its responsibility to improve, monitor, and protect public health systems, the federal government influences the healthcare market. Federal agencies influence research and technological trajectories of health care and public health.

Many factors and forces at the national level such as reimbursement schemes and regulatory policies do not support patient-centered care or high-reliability health care organizations as a whole. Although the federal government is positioned to influence change, private-sector health organizations, associations, and state governments are best positioned to experiment with mechanisms and incentives to improve the reliability of care and create healthier populations.[35]

Global

Health issues have always been global, interdependent, and diverse. Today, they are more rapid, opportunistic or threatening. Global health as a term of reference has become more common in recent years. Global health encompasses most of that which is relevant to health, including sustainable development, diseases cross international borders, factors affect public health systems globally, and the interconnectedness of health matters around the globe. Global health trends, policies on trade and travel, globalization and the "internet of things," have increased transparency and media sensationalism, and the recognition interdependency across the border have magnified global health opportunities and threats. With internet-based business, cross-border health agreements (e.g. pharmaceuticals), push back on divisive habits such as smoking, ease of international medical tourism, rapid spread of naturally occurring disease (i.e., Ebola or Zika), and the ability to concoct disease laden weapons, experts have recognized the need for active global health diplomacy and security.

Global health combines the concepts of international health, public health, to derive a definition of global health. Transnational emphasizes the critical need for collaboration and action across national boundaries. Global health builds on national public health efforts and institutions. Global health is concerned with health improvement and sustainable development, whether population-wide or individually based across all sectors, not just the area of health as systems a systems approach to assure sustainable implementation.[47] More specifically, collaboration emphasizes the critical importance of thinking through the complexity of challenges various institutions face when finding solutions. Transnational (or cross national) refers to the involvement of two or more countries that transcend national boundaries to address opportunities or counter the effects of global health issues. Research implies the importance of developing the evidence-base for policy based on a full range of disciplines especially research on the effects of transnational determinants of health. Action emphasizes the importance of evidence-based information constructively achieve health equity. Promoting (or improving) implies the importance of using a full range of public health and health promotion strategies to improve health, including those directed at the underlying social, economic, environmental and political determinants of health. Health for all refers to multi-sectoral approaches to health improvement and the need to strengthen preventive and primary health care as the basis of all health systems.[47,48]

Global health systems thinking is based on the idea health problems should address systemically rather than viewing each part in isolation. Such an approach means considering the place, and plan, they are often unpredictable and may not yield positive results all the time. From systems a thinking perspective, it is often best to facilitate an environment where local people and communities self-organize to improve health, leading to sustainable results and longer term improvements in health outcomes.

Importance of Systems Thinking and Integration

In this discussion, systems thinking requires leaders to set boundary conditions for the various levels but beware of the interactions and influences. At one extreme, there's a risk a narrow analysis misses important connections; at the other extreme, there's a system thinking approach that gets so "cross-boundary" it cannot decide what to leave out, becomes unwieldy, and faces paralysis. Systems thinking about health systems will help leaders see the critical elements of the system in question, and identify the likely unintended effects of adjustments. An intervention is typically conducted on a particular element of the system.[19] Similarly, systems thinking about health policy suggests poor health outcomes can spring from surrounding systems or social determinants of health. Therefore health organizations offer limited opportunities for improving health outcomes unless they engage in a systems approach.

Reflection

From this discussion of the levels and need for integration of health systems, what emerges is an understanding of the health systems interdependence, as networks of networks or systems of systems. This observation involves an enormous number of independent stakeholders and interests, layered by the organization, specialty, state, and national levels. If the system is approached by deconstructing the elements of the system, designing how each element should function, and reconstituting the overall system, sustainable solutions will not be generated.

The complexity of the entire health system and its role within national and global systems should be embraced. Thus health system improvement and strengthening must be approached in a different way and from a different point of view—beginning with viewing the current fragmented health systems around the world as complex adaptive heath systems and work towards integration and ultimately an interconnected global system of health and well-being for all.

PART II: METHODS AND TOOLS

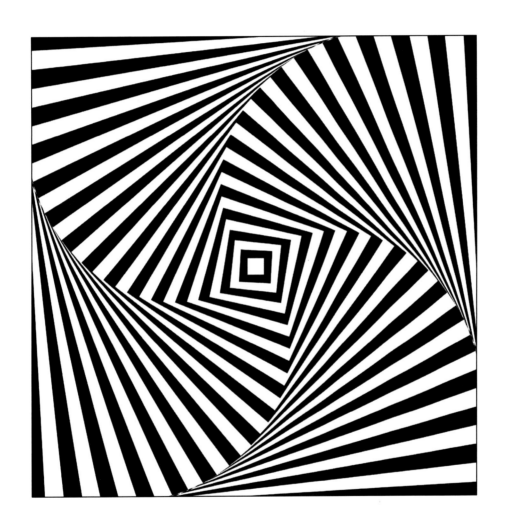

Overview of Part II

Given the health system's role in the health, wellness, resilience, and prosperity of a nation, evidence suggests a systems approach to improved integration, reliability, and health must be a priority. Health systems are complex with interconnected elements, yet too often treated as isolated and linear production units. The chronic failures (learning opportunities) in many parts of the system, such as preventable deaths and disability, underscore the need to analyze, design, and implement sustainable solutions and policies. This approach compels systems thinking for better health to include integrating the Triple Aim and the social determinants of health. The goal is to create better public and community health systems, both locally and globally. Current decision approaches are too simplistic for the health system's known and unknown dynamics. Unfortunately, this has led to well-intentioned decisions with unintended consequences, organizational resistance, and a downward spiral to complacency.[49] PART II explores Systems Thinking (ST) and System Dynamics (SD) concepts and followed by methods and tools with examples to achieve better health outcomes as defined by health leaders, organizations, and policy makers.[49] A beginning is to change how health leaders frame and analyze complex problems within health delivery, public health, community, and global health settings. There is a need to apply holistic, adaptive and integrative by concentrating on the sub-systems and their behaviors. For example, the opiate addiction crises has resulted in missed opportunities, unintended consequences of previous decisions and isolated actions taken within one part of the system thus causing negative effects in other parts of the system. This current formidable challenge will be discussed further in later chapters.

System Dynamics assumes problematic situations arise from dynamic and complex systems. Systems Thinking and particularly System Dynamics methods and tools can be applied to achieve desirable health outcomes, often without major disruptions to other parts of the system. Systems are constructed as complex networks of feedback loops with time delays and non-linear relationships. For example, patient safety is a prominent theme in health care delivery, yet the number of deaths due to preventable errors has not changed much since 2001. While leaders have embraced the magnitude of this failure in the form of "preventable harm," the leadership competencies to include application of a systems approach to sustainable solutions has not been widely applied. These situations tend to be important sources of dynamic complexity, friction, dysfunctional processes, and resistance, especially if leaders and planners not adept at recognizing dysfunctions.[49] To address these challenges and opportunities, PART I provided an overview of ST and its foundation and related theories. PART II now coupling ST and SD provide.an array of mapping systems and a series of feedback loops, translating the maps into rigorous simulation models, and analyzing future scenarios along with consequences of decisions and courses of action. SD interventions could include analysis to counter infectious disease spread, effectiveness of preventive care screening programs, waiting times for access to care, and design of adaptive primary care systems. Since health care systems exhibit high levels of dynamic complexity, these methods and tools could be used to design or implement effective policies and strategic initiatives.[49]

Chapter 5: Identification of the Characteristics and Concepts of Complex Systems

Introflection

The current US health system is a patchwork of the 1900s industrial era of public health, sanitation, and safety crises, creation of health insurance as a wage ceiling workaround during World War II, creation of Medicare and Medicaid, and American values of capitalism. It is a complex adaptive heath system characterized by non-linear paths of dysfunctional causality, feedback loops, and delays.

After numerous policy patches over the years, following the turbulent 1990s managed care era, in 2008, the Patient Protection and Affordability Care Act (PPACA) also known as the Affordable Care Act or more simply ACA, promised to transform the health system and improve it's perfromance. According to James Johnson, in the recent book *Health Organizations: Theory, Behavior, and Development*, transformational leadership, complexity management and systems thinking are required and indeed urgent.[15] To transition the complex and all too often unsafe, unreliable, costly, wasteful, unsustainable, and frustrating US health system into the most reliable health system with the healthiest population in the world, leaders at all levels will need to become systems thinkers. These policies and actions (of different stakeholders) often generate counterintuitive and unpredictable effects, sometimes long after policies have been implemented. For too long, health system problems have generally been treated as if they could simply be broken down into parts to be solved rather than understood as complex adaptive health systems. To go from where we are to a future that is much more desirable requires an understanding of the whole system and systems dynamics among its myriad components.

Transforming Health Systems

Health systems leaders must become adept at the application of agile, adaptive, and systems thinking competencies, with the goal of creating an aspirational new reality. As shown in Figure 7 below, leaders tend to respond to events and symptoms rather than seeking underlying patterns of dysfunctionality and opportunities. While most leaders do in fact look for patterns and trends, many fail to understand the underpinning structure and dynamics across the system, especially at the local level in the community or region. Instead of "fire-fighting", leaders should be better at assuming ambiguity in situations, identifying and anticipating trends, and seeking opportunitues to redesign or transform the health system. This approach includes integration of the health system across orgnizational stovepipes and throughout the community using the Triple Aim and social determinants of health as a practical framework for systems thinking.

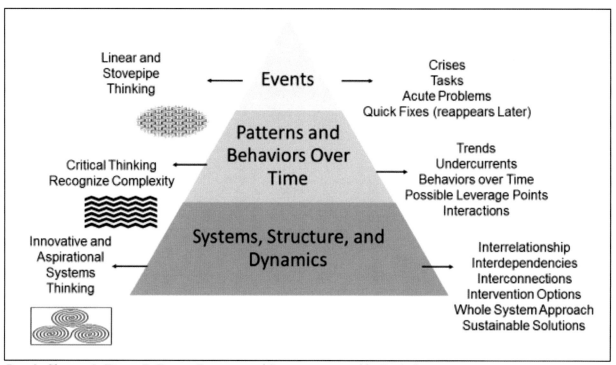

Part 2, Chapter 5, Figure 7: Events, Patterns, and Structure, created by D. Anderson

Health systems thinkers must consider three "inters:" Interactions of components within a process (i.e., heart surgery, sanitation systems), interrelationships of processes within a system (i.e., healthcare, public health, community health personalized preventive care), and interdependencies between systems and across time (i.e., community health systems integration, global health, medical tourism). Proactive health systems thinkers search for archetypes or mental models to identify functional and dysfunctional characteristics of systems: self-stabilizing, goal-seeking, self-programming, program-following, anticipatory, environment modifying, self-replicating or self-maintaining sometimes leading to organizational pathologies. Complicating this reality is a diverse set of stakeholders representing diverse interests at all levels of the system.

Common Characteristics and Behaviors

The current health system is malfunctioning because it is a managed like an assembly line and not a living and thinking system. As a result the wrong diagnosis of the characteristics and behaviors with incorrect treatment is applied. The ongoing complexity of health system transformation is the new normal today. Leaders and policy makers think (erroneously) they can manage cost by constraining one system input—money—while root causes of poor outcomes remain unaffected or exacerbated.

By contrast, systems thinkers mentally imagine a system as a series or set of feedback loops. Systems thinkers visualize possible outcomes and scenarios such as fixes that fail. To begin understanding the characteristics of complex systems should begin with understanding the characteristics and behaviors of these systems. Doing so, will result in taming "wickedness" of the health system to create the most reliable health system with the healthiest population (e.g.

better health, wellness, and resilience) in the world. As such, leaders and health policy makers must be able to identify the common characteristics and behaviors of complex systems:

Self-Stabilizing: The first characteristic of complex systems is their ability to remain stable despite ever-changing environmental conditions, inducements, and incentives. Today's health system is unstable. According to the Institute of Medicine (IOM) American health care is falling short on dimensions of quality, outcomes, costs, and equity, esepecially patient safety. Knowledge and best practices are rarely applied to improve the care processes and information generated by the care experience is too rarely shared.[50-52,53] The "wicked" nature—complex, unsafe, unreliable, costly, wasteful, unsustainable, and frustrating—of the US health system is begging for better strategic leadership and a systems approach to creating more stability leading to better health outcomes.[53-55] To achieve stability, complex systems need to consist of a great number of negative feedback loops and need to be able to obtain and use significant amounts of information about their environment. A simple system, like a thermostat, has only one loop and needs only one bit of information (room temperature) to function properly, but it can only do one job and no more. Complex health systems, on the other hand, contain thousands of simple feedback loops so they can maintain stability in the face of the many changes occur in the world.[2]

Goals: Complex systems tend to have goals and pursue those goals actively. The US health system is heavily fixated on cost, quality, and access to care. While innovation has emerged as key component, this "iron triangle" has treated each goal as separate or as an either/or proposition. While the Triple Aim attempts to create better integration of population health, experience of care, and reduced cost per capita, the goals seem health services delivery specific and not truly focused on health determinants or quality of life in the community. At the global level, the foci for the United States -- cost, quality, safety, access, integration, preventive health, productivity and outcomes -- indicates the United States may be seeking the wrong goals such as not investing in social services nor inlcuding the impact of the social detiments of health. The world health report card results, reflect an unsustainable system weakening the nation's economic, health security, and global standing. This problem requires an expansion of the health care delivery model from a purely biomedical focus with a community health, psychosocial and epidemiological ecosystem perspective. The real goal should be creating health, wellness, and resilience for the nation's citizens and a national strategic imperative.[52,56]

Policy or Program-Following: Unless intervention is achieved, complex systems tend to follow a sequence of steps or programs to achieve goals regardless of changes in the environment or new ideas for improvement at various levels. They have an innate ability to follow steps, one after another, and realize their completion using checked or unchecked feedback in any form. For example, patients have been trained to go to the doctor's office because they are not feeling well. The physician or other clinician first looks for a fever, and if there is a fever, they might look to see if there's a sore throat. If the individual has a sore throat, the clinician will probably take a throat culture to see what is causing the infection. If, however, individuals have no fever or sore throat, the clinician will follow a different path of investigation until the cause of the illness is found.[2] Ultimately the result is a paid visit with an unhealthy outcome. However, this costly and time-consuming visit possibly could have been accomplished on-line, with a less expensive professional, or other self-help resources.

Self-Reprogramming: The more complex the system, the better its ability to follow complex programs and to modify those programs so as to avoid repeating errors. For example, High Reliability Organizations (HRO) operate in complex, high-hazard domains for extended periods without serious accidents or catastrophic failures. The concept of high reliability should be attractive for health leaders, due to the complexity of operations and the risk of significant and even potentially catastrophic consequences when failures occur in health care. Reprogramming to avoid repeating mistakes is one of the most fundamental concepts in learning. If taken to the next level, a self-reprogramming system will eventually invent new, better ways to achieve the desired goal.[2] Unfortunately, many health professionals interpret high reliability as meaning effective standardization of health care processes. However, the principles of high reliability go beyond standardization. They call for standardization of routine processes so customized services or protocols can be easily adapted to human being's needs.

Anticipation: The ability to anticipate changes in the environment is the next characteristic of a complex system. In some systems, anticipation is a natural reaction. Learning from incidents becomes part of the culture. Using HROs as the setting, if health professionals adopted high reliability organization principles such as persistent mindfulness within an organization and cultivated resilience by relentlessly prioritizing safety over production minded performance pressures preventable errors may decrease. A classic example is of the military aircraft carrier: despite significant production pressures (aircrafts take off and land every 48–60 seconds), constantly changing conditions, and hierarchical organizational structure, all personnel consistently prioritize safety and have both the authority and the responsibility to make real-time operational adjustments to maintain safe operations as the top priority. Also, anticipation might be the result of insight into how the new situation will occur. In this case, the system can anticipate the response accordingly.[2]

Environment Modifying: Another option is to modify the environment to make it easier to deal with. All systems have an effect on their environment, however, it is sometimes unintentional and sometimes harmful.[2] The US health system is only beginning to focus more on a culture of health to include incorporation of the social determinants of health to create healthier communities. For example, the US health system is now starting to address social determinants of health and individual behavioral modification to create better health. This is underscored by the fact the impact on the US economy for seven preventable chronic diseases is estimated to be $1.3 trillion annually.[57] Lost worker productivity due to health is $225 billion.[58,59] Lost productive time due to health-related issues closely linked to chronic illnesses costs employers $225.8 billion per year ($1685/employee per year). If the US continues on the current trajectory, spending more than any other nation in the world and enjoying unsafe, unreliable, and mediocre health outcomes, the system could implode.[60-62]

Self-Replicating: Another quality of many complex systems is the ability to reproduce or replicate themselves. Biological reproduction or DNA is the most common, and possibly the most complex to analyze as it entails action all of the way down to the nucleus of cells. Self-replication can also occur in social systems as when a community sends representatives to a new land to form another community, or when the owner of a fast food restaurant opens another. It is important to note, however, the replicated entity, whether an urgent care center or public health system is never exactly like the first one. This indicates the complex system's ability to modify their programs slightly or adapt as a complex health system.[2]

<u>Self-Maintaining and Repairing</u>: In systems such as biological and social ones, self-maintenance and repair are built-in. While some machines are designed to self-maintain and self-repair, it is not as common a characteristic. The most obvious example of this is when an individual cuts them self or breaks a bone, the body is programmed to repair the damage. As with self-replicating systems, however, the repaired part will never exactly replicate the original. Social systems are functioning properly also self-maintain and repair. If a tornado comes to town and tears down all of the homes in a specific area, the community will eventually rebuild. The new area might not be exactly the same as the original, but it will function as before.[2]

<u>Self-Reorganizing</u>: Some complex systems also have the ability to reorganize themselves to meet new conditions or achieve new goals. Many types of living systems are capable of reorganizing themselves also, but to a more subtle extent. For instance, in response to rigorous exercise, bodies develop stronger muscles, a healthier heart, and bigger lungs.[2] However, actions taken at one time and in one subsystem have ripple effects in other systems and downstream over time. A contrast between the application of systems thinking and the more common linear approach is instructive to illustrate subtle negative effects in the health system. Cutting funds for asthma prevention programs is an action taken in the economic system causing effects in the medical system, i.e., more acute asthma and more hospital admissions, increasing expenses (back to economic system) thus self-reorganizing. Resulting school absences would reduce school performance (education system) and also would require the parent to take off work, losing his/her job (economic system) negatively impacting productivity (national system) thus more pressure on the unemployment system. Over time, increased unemployment and lack of education increases crime (social system).[1]

<u>Self-Programming</u>: Where self-reprogramming is the modification of programs in order to avoid repeating mistakes, self-programming is the development of new goals. A complex system has the ability to invent new goals and create new programs for achieving those goals. Sometimes they have similar situations to model themselves after, but usually these new goals come with an empty slate and the program devised comes from insight and ingenuity. Such an example of this is the development of the chronic disease program -- the Apollo moon landing (and now the Eliminate Cancer Moonshot) initiative, something never before achieved, was successful due to insightful and ingenious goals.[2]

Reflection

Americans would be best served by a health system to deliver reliable performance and better health constantly. Not understanding the characteristics and behaviors of a complex health system undermines the current performance. Recent estimates indicate patient safety outcomes have become worse. The Institute of Medicine (IOM) has stated, "as many as 98,000 patients deaths per years are preventable."[63,64] Ten years later, IOM reports the number of preventable deaths has not changed.[53] Unfortunately, these are not the features describing safe, quality, and accessible healthcare in America today. The US health services industry lags behind many sectors on the ability to meet patients' specific needs (e.g., access, choice, affordability) or to learn how to deliver better care, better health, and reduce per capita costs.[53]

      Today, healthcare and public health organizations can no longer afford to work in isolation, engage in linear thinking, and rely on centralized control to "fix" the health system. They must begin to reframe the conversation to create a culture of health and wellness. Application of systems thinking is a start. A redesigned health system must be seamless, transparent, and integrated with the local community. Systems thinking is a journey, not an end. Health leaders at all levels must catalyze communities of solutions and agencies across the nation. The communities of solutions must design and implement a multi-dimensional strategy – an epic campaign – to transform the health system to a model of health wellness, and resilience. For example, a systems approach to Substance Use can be used to develop recommendations for a local and national treatment strategy. The recommendations could result in sustainable solutions to improving accessibility, quality and range of substance use services and support a national strategic imperative to improving the health of the nation. This transformational effort can be accomplished within a generation of leaders only if it becomes a national strategic imperative of the highest order.[65] Health system planners and decision-makers need to recognize the nature of the system's interacting parts, define the results they really want; and, and apply the concepts and characteristics using an analytic framework. A start would be to understand and employ the right systems thinking models and tools for the appropriate situation.

Chapter 6: Methods, Models, and Tools

Introflection

Methods and tools to include models and modeling in systems thinking are designed to address complex problems, especially in the initial stages at the conceptual level. For example, many of the challenges in global health, specifically health security or sustainable development are recognized as complex health systems not simply a set of westernized healthcare templates for implementation. These approaches have resulted in limited success. A systems approach, especially systems analysis will also involve multiple interacting agents at all levels.

Systems analysis is the act of applying a systems approach. The systems approach to intervention requires leaders to see the patterns of interactions and interrelations connected with a problem. For example, organizational growth and change in one part of the system impact other areas of the system. When using the systems approach to intervention leaders must look at the pieces of the whole. Given the inter-professional approach to the delivery of health care or community health services, it is easy to see why professionals need to discuss the broader to application of systems thinking.

Systems thinking models and frameworks are widely applicable. Systems thinking involves a broad range of theories. These are rational sets of ideas or principles designed to explain something. Methods associated with systems thinking are used to investigate complex problems and processes. Systems thinking uses a broader set of methods and tools such as hardware and software used to conduct experiments, make observations, collect, organize and analyze data. While there is not consistently across the professions applying health systems thinking, the continuum of methods and tools fit into general categories.

Methods, Models, and Tools Help Leaders Sort through Messy Problems

Most health organizations are increasingly more complex. The problems they face do not exist in isolation but relate to something else in the organization or the communities they serve. Health leaders tend to react to events and respond to patterns of behavior superficially. However, deeper levels of understanding structures, processes, and relationships are needed. A lack of awareness and training on identifying and dysfunctional structures typically creates a victim mentality. Structures are not hidden, they are not obvious. Systems thinking methods, models, and tools are ways to uncover, see and understand them. Once health leaders become aware of these dysfunctional structures, how to look for them, and know them, they become readily apparent.[36] Examining a problem in isolation tends to create biased solutions affects other parts of the system. Therefore, health leaders must take precautions such as being mindful of systemic causes and effects and being more inclusive within and outside the organization for sustainable solutions.[36]

Problems tend to be messy or complex. Because problems involve many facets and organizations are made of many sub systems and linked to communities, health leaders need to understand other individual's perspectives to see different possibilities. Rather than be focused on things, relationships throughout the systems become more important. Healthy organizations are now bred from healthy relationships.[36,66,14]

The systems approach to sorting through challenging complex problems and their associated interventions eliminates biased decisions, unintended consequences, and invisible third order effects. Systems thinking must encourage leaders to look at the whole of something, not just the fragmented pieces. Unlike fragmented, i.e. Newtonian, approaches, health leaders and policymakers must study the interaction and relations of the parts as they pertain to the whole. Responsibilities in organizations are typically organized into stovepipes, specific roles, and summarized on organizational charts. Knowledge areas have separate disciplines and subjects. Schools have walled off spaces. Health and non-health leaders have been taught to think within the boundaries of these lines rather than see the opportunities outside the lines.[14]

Categories Methods, Models, and Tools

Systems tools can be divided into two broad categories: hard and soft methods and tools. In analyzing systems, two broad approaches have emerged as "engineering" and "management" driven. The engineer tends to analyze and design new systems with well-defined or "hard" methods. The manager, researcher and policy analyst uses qualitative and collaborative or "soft" methods. The application of systems thinking involves addressing problems or opportunities of significance at the organization, community, or national levels utilizing tools and techniques to bridge both approaches.

Hard methods are considered traditional ways and means of viewing and solving systems problems. These approaches--systems analysis, systems engineering, operations research-- assume an objective reality of systems being considered, a clear problem exists, and technical factors and scientific approaches to problem-solving are a priority. Hard system tools comprise Quality, Function, Deployment Diagrams, Functional Decomposition models; Integrated Definition (IDEF), Functional Flow Block Diagram, Universal Modeling Language (UML), and a broad range of modeling and statistical tools.[67]

Soft system problems typically contain fuzzy, unstructured, and ambiguous requirements. Soft systems assume organizational problems are messy or poorly defined. Stakeholders interpret problems differently. Soft methods address human factors, creativity, and intuition to solve problems or develop strategies. In many cases, the outcomes of learning and better understanding rather than a solution are the most important. Soft methods include Peter Checkland's Soft System Methodology and traditional analysis tools such as Responsibility, Accountability, Consulting, Informed (RACI) Matrixes and Swim Lane Charts.[24]

Systems thinking practitioners utilize methods and tools from both categories, however distinguishing the difference is important. Hard methods and hard instruments are rigid techniques and procedures designed to provide unambiguous solutions to well-defined data and processing problems such as waiting times and frustration levels. Soft methods are used at the discretion of the analyst who is focused on improvements to organizational or system-wide problems using concepts and creativity.

Many practitioners agree soft methods provide significant insight into broad problem definition and actor or stakeholder opinions, while hard methods provide quantitative evaluations, isolated solutions, and metrics for success. The integration of the approaches requires creativity and flexibility. For example, soft methods provide better insight into problems allowing for a more precise follow-on application of hard systems design and development. Both approaches fall into the systems thinking toolbox. Applied systems thinking provides the intersection or overlap between the two methods.[67] Often there is confusion about the value or importance of hard versus soft methods. It is not necessary to be precise about the relationship between hard and soft systems methods. It is important the systems thinker leverage both methods for the right problem with the right set of player. Doing so provides a new power for the application of systems thinking in a variety of healthcare and public health settings.[67]

Table 2
Methods, Models, and Tools

Name	Purpose and Description With Example
Agent-based modeling (ABM)	Purpose and Description: Used to create simulated or visuals representations of complex systems. Models individual agents (i.e., actors and stakeholders) who interact with each other and the environment. Although the interactions or non-interactions based on simple, pre-defined rules, in a complex system ABM allows for identification of gaps, emergent behaviors, underlying patterns, and relationships leading to improved policies, processes, or services. Example: Study incentives with Accountable Care Organization (ACO) agents: payers, providers, and patients to share risk, payment, and savings for congestive heart failure (CHF) procedures.[68]
Network Analysis (or Social Network Analysis)	Purpose and Description: Uses graphical methods to analyze relations between nodes. Social network analysis applies network theory to social entities (e.g., individuals, groups, organizations) to understand nodes (individual actors within a network), and interrelations (the type of relationships) between actors and stakeholders. Example: While progress on understanding networks, structures, and development has been made, little is known about the effectiveness on their contributions to the quality of care and patient safety. According to a synthesis of 29 published articles, evidence of health care workforce's social networks reveal insights and effects on adoption and coordination of strategic initiatives.[69]
Scenario Planning or Futuring	Purpose and Description: Integrative strategic planning method uses tools to identify and analyze possible future events, possible alternative outcomes, and actionable insights. Can involve quantitative projections and qualitative judgments about alternative futures. The real value lies in learning from the process than the actual scenarios.

Name	Purpose and Description With Example
	Example: Scenario planning was used to focus on high-impact, uncertain driving forces affecting the field of radiology.[70]
Systems Dynamics Modeling	Purpose and Description: A multi-varied approach uses tools to understand the behavior of complex systems over time. Methods include stocks and flows and feedback loops designed to solve problems and assess impacts of changing variables over small periods of time while allowing for feedback and various interactions and delays. Example: The Centers for Disease Control and Prevention (CDC) sponsored development of a systems dynamics model of diabetes prevalence and complications to be used for designing and evaluating intervention strategies. The model can be utilized by other public health stakeholders for policy analysis and strategic planning at the national, state, and local levels.[71]
Participatory Impact Pathways Analysis (PIPA)	Purpose and Description: PIPA, a workshop-based involving stakeholders combines impact pathway logic models and network mapping to create clarity of complexity and sustainable solutions. PIPA workshops help participants uncover assumptions and underlying mental models about how projects or policies should be developed and implemented. Example: A case assessed threats of emerging infectious disease: Avian Influenza to Ebola resulting from of complex social and ecological interactions in Africa. This case examined the dynamics of disease and consequences of poverty and social justice. The process facilitated the design of policies to identify pathways to improve health for the poor and inform policy institutions and field practitioners.[72]
Causal Loop Diagrams (CLD)	Purpose and Description: CLDs produce qualitative illustrations of mental models, focused on causality and feedback loops. Feedback loops can be reinforcing or balancing. CLDs explain the role of such loops within a system. Example: In many countries, health systems expenditures have increased; pressures on affordability and accessibility in Singapore's health system are mounting. CDLs were used to elucidate complexities brought about by multiple interconnected subsystems and their complex relationships.[73]
Stock And Flow Diagrams	Purpose and Description: Stock and flow diagrams are quantitative system dynamics tools used for illustrating a system can be used for model-based policy analysis in a simulated, dynamic environment. Stock and flow diagrams explicitly incorporate feedback to understand complex system behavior and capture non-linear dynamics. Example: Extensive use of systems dynamics tools including Stock and flow diagrams, CLDs, and systemigram to uncover barriers to health,

Name	Purpose and Description With Example
	sanitation, nutrition in rural Georgia. The workshop series resulted in the major players understanding the impacts of the causes and effects of actions and decisions on each other throughout the system. When everyone could see clearly how their different goals and incentives had led to fragmented and piecemeal efforts strategic and holistic approach to improving disparities followed.[74]
Process Mapping Or Diagraphs and Systemigrams	Purpose and Description: Tools such as flow charts to provide pictorial representations of a sequence of actions and responses. Their use can be flexible, such clarity of current processes and identify bottlenecks, constraints, or inefficient steps to produce an "As-Is" versus "To-Be" map or visual. Example: A sequential and a hierarchical process map of a community-based anticoagulation clinic was produced using interview results, walk-throughs, training sessions, and review of protocols and policies. The study concluded evidence exists organization of information in an external representation affects better decision-making.[75]
Systems Archetypes	Purpose and Description: Systems archetypes are mental models used to describe behaviors and patterns between parts of a system. These models provide mental templates to illustrate behaviors with balancing and reinforcing feedback loops. Archetypes can be used by teams to diagnosis how a system is working or not working and how performance changes over time. Example: Archetypes helped hospital leaders recognize patterns of behavior already present in their organizations. They served as a means to gain insight into underlying systems structures, uncover fallacies in strategic thinking, and defy fallacies during policy or strategic initiatives implementation.[76]

Adapted by D. Anderson from Peters DH. The Application of Systems Thinking in Health: Why Use Systems Thinking? Health Research Policy and Systems 2014

Aligning Problems with Methods, Models, and Tools in Health Settings

Systems thinking tools have been applied in a wide variety of settings: global health, public and community health, and health settings. In most cases, the methods can be replicated in any of the other settings. For example, Bishai et al. present a simple systems dynamics model using stocks and flow and causal loops diagrams to illustrate the trade-off effects and unintended consequences of policy choices related to allocation to preventive and curative services.[77] In this simulation, disease A, a curable disease can be shortened by curative care. Curative care workers are financed by public spending and private fees to cure disease. Disease B, a fatal but preventable disease is prevented with non-personal, preventive services delivered by public health workers supported solely by public spending. Each worker attempts to tilt the balance of government expenditures towards their interests. The model demonstrated the effects of lost disability-adjusted life years and costs over the course of several epidemics of each disease. Policy interventions were tested. The model illustrated spending more on curing disease a leads paradoxically to a higher overall disease burden of unique cases of disease B. This paradoxical behavior can be stopped by eliminating lobbying, fees for curative services and blocking public health funding. The underlying dynamics resemble features of a US health system centered disease-specific curative programs like HIV/AIDS or malaria rather than focusing on population-level prevention services and surveillance.[77]

Some tools are applied to facilitate groups of individuals, so a common understanding of an issue will prompt further synthesis, inquiry, and action. For example, "systems archetypes" are common and usually reoccurring patterns of behavior in organizations, sometimes invisible or ignored. These patterns usually result in negative consequences. Systems archetypes can help teams proactively understand generic patterns of interaction applicable to their story with templates and other structured tools.

Archetypes can also be used more proactively as planning tools. By looking ahead at possible systemic consequences of proposed actions, leaders must identify structures impeding and advancing progress. Using archetypes in this way can help potential problems and opportunities surface so teams can ahead of the power curve. For example, in a series of case studies dissertation, *Developing a System Resilience Approach to the Improvement of Patient Safety in National Health System (NHS) Hospitals,* five versions of Peter Senge's archetypes are illustrated: safe practice, drift, tip, collapse and transition towards failure. The objective was to explore how a systems approach can be used to provide insight into patient safety issues in England's National Health Service (NHS) hospitals. The archetypes through balancing, reinforcing, and vicious feedback loops illustrated as hospitals became overcrowded, complexity increased and risk to patient safety and harm increased. This case reinforced the need for the possibilities of applying systems thinking and what constitutes system resilience, will assist policy makers to create conditions for greater adaptability by front line staffs to avoid patient harm.

In addition to systems archetypes, **Causal Loop Diagrams (CLD)** are created without templates and involve drawing an understanding of how elements of a problem are related to each other. They usually begin as descriptions or feedback loops outlining how one thing causes another in either a positive or negative direction.[78] Typically, feedback loops are identified between the different elements of a system. These loops can be reinforcing or positive: A produces more B, then B produces more A such as a vicious cycle of malnutrition and infections. The loops can be balancing or negative feedback loops, where a positive change in one loop leads to pushing back in the opposite direction such as when increasing body temperature produce sweating, which in turn cools down the body.[78]

The elements of a **CLD** might be converted into a quantitative systems dynamics model by classifying the elements as "Stocks, Flows, And Rates" by equations to describe the relationships between individual variables. For example, **stocks** could be the accumulation patient populations such as patients calling the appointment desk or waiting to be seen. **Flows** are rates at which populations enter and depart a medical clinic or from the time they make an appointment to the time they pick up a medication. Flows change the levels of stocks such as rates patients arrive at check-in. Stocks flows, and **rates** can be directly translated into set models for simulation of options to improve flow.

Some tools are used to map out events or how processes are connected. **Network Mapping, Social Network Analyses, and Process Mapping** involve several tools to analyze connections between individuals, organizations, or processes. Network analysis has been used by public health leaders to study disease transmissions such as HIV/AIDS and other sexually transmitted diseases. Information transmission, diffusion of innovation, the role of social support, assessing the influence of social networks on health behavior change has been applied in numerous settings.[79] As a global health example, Malik et al. mapped out the network of actors involved in physician's seeking advice in Pakistan. Using measles and tuberculosis as examples, the study examined the advice-seeking behavior of primary health care (PHC) physicians in Pakistan. The results indicated the absence of a functioning patient referral system limited effective communication between PHC and higher levels of care.[80]

A flow chart is one of the more common tools used to draw a process or a system. For example, Goulet et al. used systems thinking tools to determine the rate of preventable patient deaths who died early and unexpectedly the following discharge from the emergency department (ED) and admitted to four Paris, France hospitals. The study concluded more than half of unexpected deaths related to preventable medical errors.[81]

Innovation History or Change Management History is used to capture the history of key events, issues, and outcomes as part of an implementation of solutions. For example, Zhang et al. looked back over the last 35 years of the development of the medical system in rural China. The history illustrated the complex and political nature of health system development and reform. The study concluded governments need to increase their capacity to analyze the health sector as a complex system and to manage change processes.[82]

Participatory Impact Pathways Analysis (PIPA) involves workshops and a combination of tools to clarify interventions or the mapping of a network. PIPAs enhance understanding through participation with beneficiaries, implementers, and stakeholders. For example, a PIPA, conducted by the Institute of Developmental Studies addressed how to build resilient health systems in case of another Ebola outbreak in West Africa. The results yielded insight on how to create resilient health systems in Nigeria and highlighted the basics of outbreak control within a larger complex adaptive systems.[83]

Agent-based modeling takes advantage of a wide variety of theories, methods, and tools to simulate the interaction of agents (e.g., actors, stakeholders, individuals or organizations) to see how real world phenomena affect the system as a whole. The models involve understanding how agents who work at different levels and with differing decision-making rules can improve processes for adaptation.[78] For example, provider behavior changes to achieve maximum financial and quality outcomes of an Accountable Care Organization (ACO) have been modeled. The results showed nonlinear provider behavior change patterns corresponding to changes in payment model designs. The outcomes vary by providers with different quality or financial priorities, and are most sensitive to the cost-effectiveness of Congestive Heart Failure (CHF) interventions ACOs implement. This study demonstrates how this method and model can inform policymakers and health leaders on important decisions such as illustrating ACOs are interdependent with payment model design, provider characteristics, and cost and effectiveness of health interventions.[68]

In public health and medicine, use research evidence on the efficacy of interventions to inform decisions with an expectation of a future effect. Systems thinking methods, models and tools such as **Scenario Planning**, can also be used to **forecast** future events. However, such methods are intended to be used for identifying possible outcomes to provide insights on how to prepare for the event rather than fixating on a specific solution or outcome.[78]

Reflection

In his landmark address on "Why Model?" Joshua Epstein at the NYU College of Global Public Health, identified 16 reasons on why we can gain from using models.[84] Most of the reasons apply to systems thinking while many specific reasons relate to being able to explain how things work. Systems thinking is particularly useful for explaining how complex systems work. Many systems thinking methods, models and tools can be used to "kick-start" problem solving, exchange ideas, and evaluate assumptions related to policy interventions in a psychologically safe setting. Agent-based models, systems dynamics, and scenario planning are particularly useful for these purposes.

The systems approach to intervention eliminates boundaries separating organizations into parts, resulting in healthier, more effective organizations. Through the use of methods, models, and tools, systems analysis focuses on causes rather than symptoms. Systems analysis discovers the reasons for the problem and fixes it. It is only then symptoms go away. Systems thinking sounds complex, but it's about creating simpler, wiser solutions. Systems thinking helps leaders recognize the basic forces working behind all actions, individuals, and problems, so time is not wasted trying to fix the symptoms of the problem to create sustainable solutions.[85] While all of these tools are valuable, common methods and tools are used extensively throughout systems thinking. These are discussed and explored in the following chapters.

Chapter 7: Fundamental Tools – Stocks, Flows, and Loops

Introflection

The range of "Tools" to be mastered before one can understand complex systems is not as enormous as one might think. In fact, it may be more intuitive than expected. The mixing-and-matching of "Tools" make up the common DNA of all systems—whether physical, biologic or social—revealing simplicity underlying the complexity of systems.

The heart of Systems Thinking is to help leaders and organizations visualize and create sustainable solutions to complex problems or better yet, build on past successes as opportunities arise, and predict the behavior of complex systems (system wide or individual). Whether the system is lamenting a sustainable development goal in a country, managing a patient-centered medical home or medical supply chain, leading a community health integration initiative, or establishing health system policies, breaking a system into its component pieces and studying the pieces separately is, thus, an inadequate way to understand the whole. Health systems leaders must see the inter-relationships, interdependencies, and interconnections. Systems thinking guides health leaders and policy makers to understand the dynamics of a situation, root causes leading to dysfunction, and assessment of perverse policies or processes at any level.

While the use of systems thinking in health settings and personal health is less widely adopted, health is precisely the setting where dynamic systems complexity is most problematic and the stakes are highest. As a specific health and personalized example to illustrate the "basics" of systems thinking, the 2010 Report by the U.S. Institute of Medicine: *Bridging the Evidence Gap in Obesity Prevention: A Framework to Inform Decision Making* declares to reduce obesity, a systems approach will be needed. As obesity continues to increase, clear solutions have not emerged. Reducing obesity poses a challenge for the health system and quality of life. It is a complex problem with many interconnections and interdependencies. The complexity of obesity challenges traditional primary care practices that have been structured to address simple or less complicated conditions. At the national policy level, obesity is clearly a complex problem for both the individual and society. However, complex problems have common characteristics at any level such as heterogeneity, nonlinearity, interdependence, and self-organization. As such problems require a different approach rather than a reductionist search for the causes. Systems thinking provides new ways to collectively address complex societal problems like obesity, where biology interacts with social, cultural and environmental factors across organizations and all levels.[86-91]

Understanding and learning to apply these "Tools" is a powerful mental model allowing leaders and policymakers to see through complexity to the deeper structures and patterns that drive (and thus help explain) complex events and phenomena. For example is human weight and energy regulation.. They are parts of a complex psychobiological system involving behavioral acts of eating, ingestion, and assimilation of food, storage, and utilization of energy and interactions with the external environment (cultural and physical). These factors are interconnected, pushing each other in dysfunctional directions. Appetite and perceptions shape body weight and body weight influences perceptions and appetite. Weight reflects activity levels and self-esteem and activity levels reflect weight.[92]

Bathtubs (Stocks)

To illustrate the basic tool sets, the reader can use a familiar example: a bathtub. Because of water, unlike energy, is something to be seen and touched, visualizing how a bathtub works is a much easier task for most individuals. Imagine observing someone filling a bathtub with water in preparation for taking a bath. Individuals who observe the process will see is this: faucet opening, water flowing, and water level rising in the figure below.

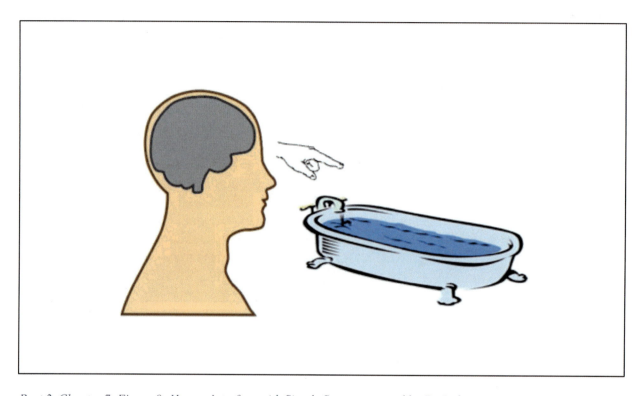

Part 2, Chapter 7, Figure 8: Human Interface with Simple System, created by D. Anderson

These processes do not tell the whole "tub-filling story." Most notably, they miss the essence of what regulates the tub-filling process, namely, the tub- filling <u>goal</u>. When and individual fills a bathtub to take a bath, they have a "desired water level" in mind—a goal. Options include plugging the drain, turning on the faucet, and watching the water level rise. As the water level rises, an adjustment to the faucet position slows the flow of water and turns it off when the water reaches the desired level. Thus, the more complete (and more accurate) a representation (or model) of what is happening looks like the figure below.

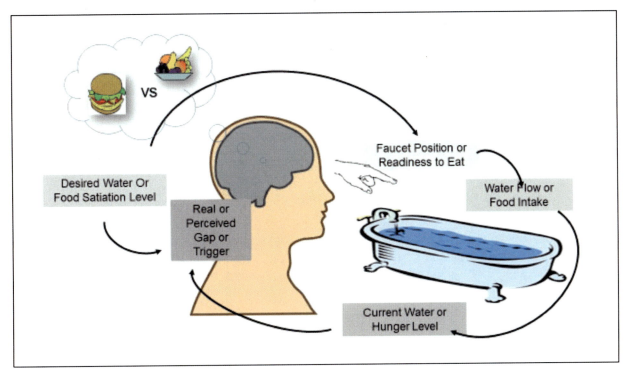

Part 2, Chapter 7, Figure 9: Human Interface with Other Systems, created by D. Anderson

Notice the goal—the "desired water level"—and the arrow-like connections (which are cause-and-effect connections) are not visible in the physical system. There is an ideal goal and discrepancy-measuring process going on in the individual's mind while manipulating the faucets. When the process is observed in daily life, it is natural to think of the faucet controlling the amount of water in the tub--unidirectional cause-and-effect of the faucet opening, water flowing, and water level rising. Further, the influence is mutual rather than one-way: the faucet's opening affects the water level <u>and</u> the water in the bathtub, through sight, action, and habits control how long the faucet is opened and when it is turned off.

This simple system demonstrates three things:

1. While individuals are inclined to think in straight lines or linear fashion, reality often works in circles or non-linear ways..
2. Learning to "see" the circular information flows within systems (e.g., the circular loop of cause-and-effect process seen in the figure is important because they are the key to regulating what is happening… in this case helping regulate water flow to fill the tub to some desired level.
3. This simple system has the basic building blocks of which all systems are made.

All systems—whether simple or complex, whether biologic, behavioral, technologic or economic—can be modeled using the fundamental or basic tool sets of systems thinking: Stocks (or bathtubs), Flows (or faucets), and Information (causal) links between them.

Bathtubs (Stocks) and Faucets (Flows)

Dynamic systems—the human body—can be modeled as stocks, flows, and rates of flow threaded together by causality or information feedback loops. Stocks flows, and rates of flow constitute the two different processes—accumulation and flow—how reality works and how systems change.

Stocks and flows should be familiar. Stocks are containers or accumulators of something. The contents increase or decrease as a function of how much "something" flows in or flows out. A bathtub is a stock with water flowing in and draining out such as a savings account or food. It is an "information" type stock in which money or food accumulates when an individual's deposits (breakfast snacks, lunch, dinner, binge eating) is greater than withdrawals (overflow of the wrong food intake). Stocks capture the "state of the system." Mathematically, they are called "state variables." Stocks are measured at one point in time such as calorie intake. Stocks start with some initial value such as hunger and after that changed only by flows into and out of them. There are no inputs immediately change stocks. Similarly, so is the body—a stock of fat accumulates the difference between energy in (from eating) and energy out (from physical activity).[86-90] Stocks can also be a source of delay in a system. Also, in healthcare or public health settings, examples of other types of stocks include:

- Individuals with different disease states (susceptible, infective, immune)
- Stockpiled vaccines and medications
- Pregnant women
- Males or females between the age of x and y or demographic, gender, nationality
- High-risk individuals by chronic disease types
- Health workers in all functional areas
- Medicine in stocks on the ward, office, or warehouse
- Blood sugar levels
- Beds in an emergency room, ICU, operating ward, or observation unit

By using the basic tool sets, health leaders, medical social scientists, and policy analysts learn why it is extremely useful to be able to discern what is a stock (bathtub) and what is a flow (faucet) in the systems they deal in successive levels of the health system. Leaders acquire a skill while in a system like a bathtub so they easily recognize situations or opportunities to control, modify or eliminate flows into and out of the bathtub. In discussing human weight and energy regulation systems individuals can make sense of the use of simple visual toolsets models look like in the figure below.

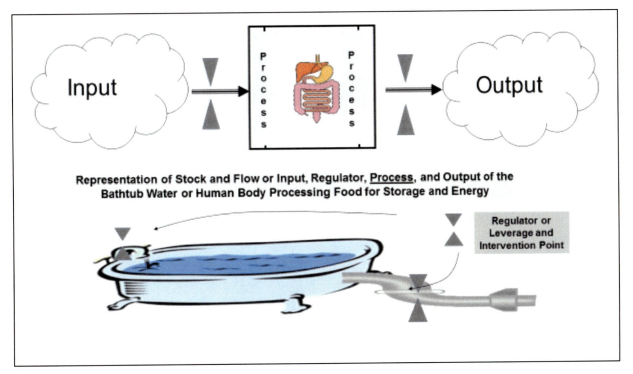

Part 2, Chapter 7, Figure 10: Simple Input, Process, and Output Model Illustrating Stocks, Flows, and Rates, created by D. Anderson

Leaders and policy analysts can represent stocks and regulators as leverage for intervention points and possibilities by rectangles—suggesting a container holding the contents of the stock. Once conceptually sound, stock and flow structures in systems of all kinds can be found. When compared to the bathtub, the level of energy stored in the human body constitutes a stock (primarily fat), with food intake as its inflow rate and energy expenditure as its outflow rate.

Flows are visuals represented with pipes and valves. Inflows are represented by a pipe (arrow) pointing into the stock, and outflows are represented by pipes pointing out of (draining or subtracting from) the stock. Further, a stock is the memory of changing flows within the system. If the outflows exceed (human energy or calories burned) the inflows, the stock (stored fat) levels decrease. If outflows equal the inflows, the stock (body weight) will not change or will be held in dynamic. For example, research demonstrates the human capacity for self-regulation. As a limited resource, self-regulation is critical for successful weight regulation. As an analogy, storage and depletion of physical energy or human capacity for self-regulation are the equivalents of a reservoir—or stock—is consumed and replenished with self-control and rest.[93] Stocks are increased by decreasing outflows. Stocks act as delay buffers or shock absorbers in systems. Stocks allow inflows and outflows to be coupled in independent.[94]

Also, stock and flow structures are not limited to physical "stuff," however. For example, research demonstrates human capacity for self-regulation is a critical factor for weight regulation. In many cases, this self-regulatory function is limited. As an analogy, storage and depletion of physical energy, the human capacity for self-regulation can be considered a reservoir—or stock—consumed and replenished with the exertion of self-control and rest.[92,95]

Information

The third basic tool illustrated in the following figure as the information (causal) link(s) in systems. In practice, these are harder to discern because they are not as visible as the bathtub and the faucet. For example, when individuals look at a system, most see the physical "stuff." Individuals see material things like tubs, water, dollar bills, and food. Causal links, on the other hand, are not physical objects, they are *relationships* between objects often times the inter-relationships and interdependencies coupled with communication.

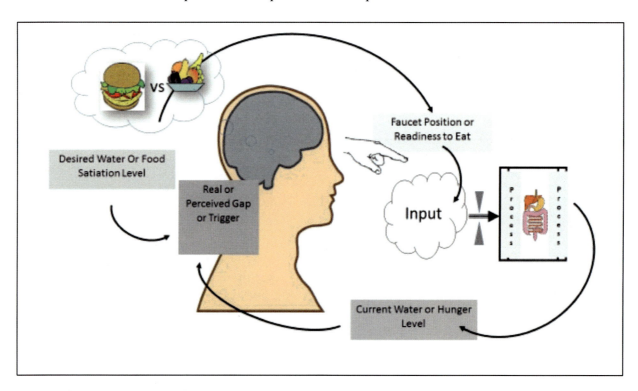

Part 2, Chapter 7, Figure 11: Illustration of Causal Links As Part of Stocks, Flows, and Rates, created by D. Anderson

Going back to the bathtub example: the physical "action" (such as faucet opening – water flowing – water level rising (or eating)) is readily observable. Less so is the information causal (something triggered an individual to reach for food when it was not necessarily needed) link: Information about the level of water in the tub causes individuals to adjust the faucet position to decrease the inflow rate and ultimately turn off the water when the level in the tub reaches the desired level. To see them take in less food requires more effort such as removal of mental blinders to see causal relationships is imperative.[89,90]

Circles or Loops

A significant feature of these causal links is they often form circles or loops — rarely do they work in one direction. In the bathtub case, the two-way interactions together form a loop. Putting the two together, loop is formed. Learning from circles and loops provides feedback on the processes to develop the skill of systems of a health systems thinker. These circular processes drive system behavior at any level — e.g., drive a system to grow and snowball such as an disease epidemic or seek to achieve and maintain some desired goal (like a person filling a bathtub or a thermostat 's set to maintain a room's temperature). Without **feedback**, it would be almost impossible for a system to achieve a desired goal or health outcome. Think about the bathtub example. If the system was as simple as depicted in figure below — with no feedback from the bathtub to the decision maker — how would individuals know when to stop filling? There won't be. Variation, physical and mental waste, and frustration or negativity sets in. Thus feedback loops are a chain of causation actions.

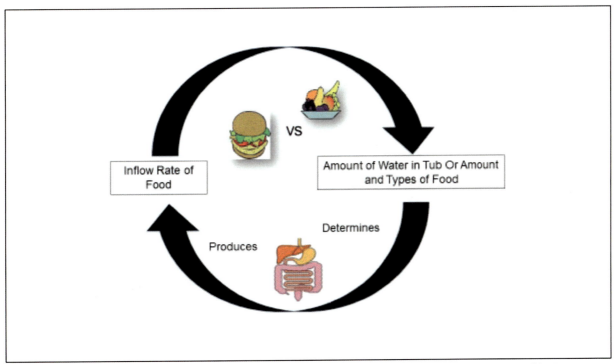

Part 2, Chapter 7, Figure 12: Circular Thinking Versus Linear Thinking in Systems Thinking, created by D. Anderson

The circular (feedback) process regulates the filling of the bathtub is not unique to bathtubs. Indeed, systems of all kinds rely on the same structure to achieve their goals. Our body (physiology) is no exception. A good example of is how the body maintains weight and core body temperature at 98.6 degrees Fahrenheit (its target). The system works almost exactly like the bathtub system above can be seen in the figure below. This figure depicts the two loops side by side: on the left is the familiar bathtub filling loop and on the right the feedback loop for regulating body temperature.

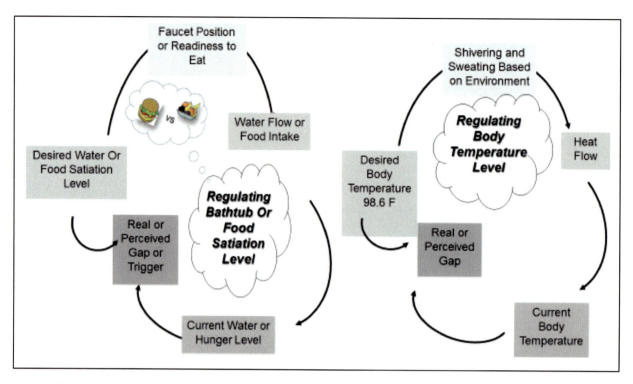

Part 2, Chapter 7, Figure 13: Illustration of Causal Links and Loops between Human Functions and Thinking, created by D. Anderson

Both work the same way. Here is how the core body temperature is regulated: If body temperature should rise—on a hot day or after a burst of physical activity—it creates a "gap" between "desired body temperature" and "actual body temperature." When sensed by the brain, the command is issued to the sweat glands to induce sweating. The evaporation of the sweat— rather than the sweating per se— would eventually cool the body down.

Furthermore, similar to the bathtub above a rise of the water level causes an adjustment to the faucet position. Eventually, it is turned off when the water reaches desired levels. The brain relies on feedback from the body (sensory information) to determine is the goal is achieved (core temperature back down to 98.6 degrees Fahrenheit) to stop the sweating. The same loop works to *raise* body temperature if it drops below the desired 98.6 degrees Fahrenheit say on a chilly night—in this case by inducing shivering. The body's feedback process regulates core body temperature serves us well because in this case the system's goal (maintaining body core temperature at 98.6 degrees Fahrenheit) works just fine for us. But what if the goals differ? What if individuals are trying to regulate each other with goal-seeking feedback processes such as peer pressure? Resistance sets in.

Because of the importance of ensuring sufficient energy for survival and reproduction, the human body has evolved feedback mechanisms to maintain its fat reserves at desired levels. Moreover, the body's feedback (also referred to as homeostatic) process aims to maintain the fat reserves is identical to the above temperature-regulating process. In a manner analogous to the rise or drop in body temperature, when significant weight is lost on a diet, the loss is interpreted by the body as a deprivation "crisis" that needs to be contained. Resistance sets in.

To restrain the rate of tissue depletion, the body compensates by slowing its metabolism (akin to the body changing its light bulbs to fluorescent lights to save energy). This process decreases total energy expenditure and shrinks the diet's energy deficit, which, in turn, (and unfortunately for the dieter) dampens the rate of weight loss. The body, in other words, "resists" intervention or dieting. Resistance occurs because well-intentioned interventions (e.g. dieting to lose weight) are at odds with the goals of the system (to maintain fat reserves), and as a result are counteracted by the system. Our bodies' wired-in feedback process to regulate (protect) its energy reserves is one reason why weight-loss strategies are rarely as straightforward as advertised. It is why weight lost tends to decline with time—even if the prescribed diet is maintained—and why individuals tend to lose less weight than they expect... much less. Balancing feedback loops for goal seeking structures and systems at any level is highly desired, especially policy levels. However, they are both sources of stability and resistance to change. Reinforcing loops are self-enhancing, leading to growth or a collapse over time. The information delivered by a feedback loop — on physical feedback — can affect the future behavior; it cannot deliver a signal fast enough to correct a group drove the back.[86-88]

Reflection

While the three goal-seeking feedback processes has been examined—filling the bathtub analogy, regulating body temperature, and maintaining fat reserves—all accomplish their "missions" in pretty much the same way. There is one significant difference between the temperature-regulating system and the other two. In the case of body temperature regulation, the "goal" (98.6 degrees) is static—it does *not* change over time; in the bathtub case and fat reserves, it often does. For example, in the case of body fat regulation, the "goal"—often referred to as the "set point"—is a moving target can ratchet up over time as a result of weight gain. Gaining a significant amount of weight can thus cause body energy reserves to be regulated at a higher set point and ultimately to "defend" the elevated body weight. The practical lesson from this is clear: Don't delay. It is crucial to arrest and then reverse weight gain before a higher set-point is wired-in.[86-90] Systems thinking gives rise to better understanding the obesity epidemic at multiple levels including community and policy levels. Actors, stakeholders, and organizations matter for the entire system to function optimally. Providing system support helps networks of individuals become communities of practice to accelerate the pace of effective action against obesity. Efforts related to isolated causes of obesity such as food deserts, inactivity on playgrounds, and targeted advertising of sugary foods, must give way to focus on solutions to effect the entire system and communities.[96] Systems thinking provides a means for health teams, health leaders, and health policy makers who are discouraged by the complexity of obesity. Approaching causes of obesity with systems thinking is essential for creating a health system that promotes innovative and collaborative practices for individuals, communities and nations dealing with obesity.

Chapter 8: Understanding Systems Dynamics

Introflection

System dynamics (SD) is an outgrowth of systems theory most notably chaos theory to understand the dynamic behavior of complex systems. Developed in the 1950s to improve understanding of complex business processes, SD can be applied in the public health and healthcare sectors to create policies to drive building healthier communities. System dynamics (SD) is an approach to understanding the nonlinear behavior of complex systems over time using stocks, flows, feedback loops, and time delays. The basis for the method recognizes the structure of any open living systems is circular and interlocking with time-delayed relationships among its parts. In many cases, this is more important in determining its behavior as the individual parts in isolation. The value of SD in the health sector is increasing. For example, SD methods to improve "end-to-end" operational aspects of health system capacity and delivery and analyze policy options to guide resolving complex public health problems. From a leadership perspective, SD lends itself to understanding different viewpoints of the main community actors and stakeholders to focus on true underlying causes of a problem and achieve consensus for action.

Current models have the ability to help assess resources and options for organizations and communities who must work with finite resources using systems thinking tools in a wide variety scenarios. For example, system dynamics modeling of chronic disease prevention could seek to incorporate the interacting elements of the social determinants of health to create a community approach to improving outcomes, reducing health, risk, and environmental factors, and optimizing health-related resources and delivery systems impacting a community, state, and national policy. System dynamics or SD is a system thinking approach to address complexity, variability, and uncertainty related to a sustainable model for health. This chapter discusses health system problems and the need to consider a sustainable approach in addressing these challenges.

Systems Dynamics and Complexity in Health Systems

As the United States continues its quest for health care reform, policymakers must use a variety of mechanisms to control health care costs and other phenomena in the environment. These mechanisms include regulations in the form of multiple feedback loops enforced through surveys, certifications, payments, and penalties—in many cases with perverse incentives or conflicting feedback loops. These, along with policy and mechanical approaches, often lead to unintended consequences such as disparities in access to care, poorer health outcomes, and increased costs each with long feedback loops, lagging information flow, or time delays. It is due to the complexity of the health care system—by its intricate design and nonlinear, dynamic, and unpredictable nature leading to major disturbances.[38]

Disturbances in health systems can also be caused by systems dynamics and complexity. To help guide future policies and minimize disturbances or unanticipated consequences of regulation, policymakers need to approach health care as a complex dynamic system and apply the principles of complexity science to achieve policy goals.[38] Understanding health system dynamics is a necessary step in understanding the underlying causes of complex problems that emerge. Given the large number of courses of action, selection may be difficult. However, decision making can be aided by the hard and soft methods, models and tools of systems thinking.

System failure is often due to a health leader's inability to recognize and manage "dynamic complexity" early and often. Leaders too often tend to approach problems in a mechanistic or linear manner. Dynamic complexity arises when:

- Short and long term consequences of the same action are dramatically different
- The effect of an action in one part of the system is entirely different from its impact on another part of the system
- Well-intentioned actions often lead to counter-intuitive, delayed, and almost invisible and results.

In contrast to mechanical systems where parts interact in a linear manner to produce predictable outputs, components of complex systems interact nonlinearly and typically produce unexpected results. Understanding dynamic complexity is a means to identify leverage points in a system to improve or and avoid resistance to policies and change. There are three drivers of dynamic systems:

1. First, multiple feedback loops are present. This driver is due to availability or non-availability of stocks, flows, and rates of the flow such as transfer of funding levels to state levels with strings and oversight responsibility for managed care services.
2. Second, time delays between the cause and effect of an action such as assuming larger co-pays and deductibles will deter overutilization only to find, delay of care, especially preventive care resulted in more complex and costly problems.
3. Third, the existence of non-linear relationships among the system's elements such as a disconnect between the delivery of curative care and the social determinants of health impacts safety, well-being, and choices of a community's population.

The output of a linear or mechanical system can be controlled by manipulating parts, while the output is dynamic thus behaving differently according to the conditions and feedback. An example, of linear thinking, is focusing on access, quality, and cost in isolation as either/or options. However, it is well-recognized natural, and human systems and health systems are combinations of multi-loop, dynamic, complex, and non-linear systems. The health care system includes networks of components: Hospitals, clinics, nursing homes, rehabilitation units, patient homes, families, and patients. These systems interact nonlinearly on different levels: patient, family, health team, medical center, community, and government. These fragmented systems tend to produce unintended consequences: adverse drug reactions, nosocomial infections, re-hospitalizations, and functional decline as a result of linear decision making.[97,98]

By using the bathtub, stocks, and flows, the figure below illustrates how the health system and creating healthier communities works. According to the World Health Organization (WHO), living conditions are the everyday environment where individuals live, play and work.

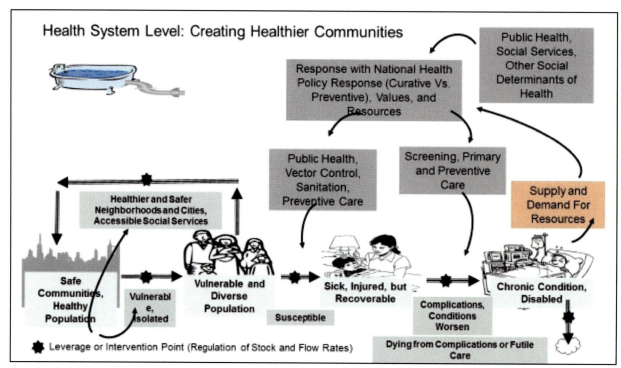

Part 2, Chapter 8, Figure 14: Understanding How to Create Healthier Communities. Adapted by D. Anderson from Milstein, B, Overview of Systems Dynamics Simulation Modeling, Systems Thinking and Modeling Workshop; 2006

These living conditions are products of social, economic, and physical circumstances all of which have an impact on personal health. Many of these factors are outside the immediate control of the individual.[99] In others words, adverse conditions include circumstances or quality of life-inhibiting an individual's freedom to live and develop their full potential. Phenomena such as hunger, war, environmental decay, homelessness, illiteracy, and injustice are examples of adverse living conditions. All of these inhibitors are related to the social determinant of health.[100]

Health Systems at all Levels Contain Multiple Feedback Loops

Every complex system is built upon two primary core elements: positive and negative feedback loops. The first step to understanding the organization of a complex system, or how it works, is to see how these two different feedback loops can be linked together to build up more complex systems.[2] Most thinking is based on the events, linear experiences, and an open loop view of the world.[101] Actions taken by an agent such as a stakeholder in a system will upset the system's equilibrium and trigger reactions from other actors to restore stability. Such thinking limits the explanation of situations, being a result of successive events linked by linear cause-effect relationships.[87,97,98,101,102]

The figure below provides some examples of feedback loops and effects. The four boxes across the bottom are the continuum of health, starting on the far left-hand side of the graph, which is where individuals are healthy and not vulnerable. The next box being where they are vulnerable, they have a risk or a social situation that makes them susceptible to diseases. Then, the individuals who have the disease, not necessarily the complications. Lastly, the individuals who are sick and have complications.

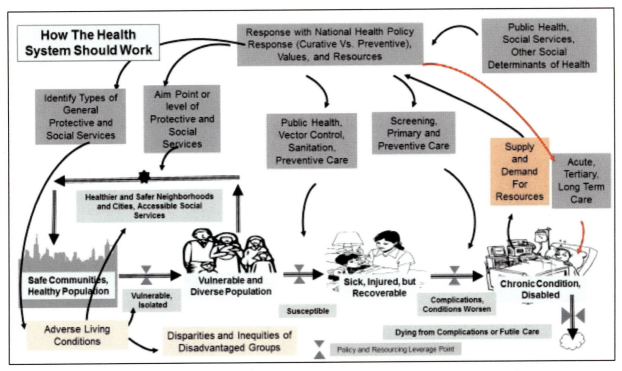

Part 2, Chapter 8, Figure 15: How the Health System Should Work Using Policy Intervention and Leverage Points. Understanding How to Create Healthier Communities. Adapted by D. Anderson from Milstein, B, Overview of Systems Dynamics Simulation Modeling, Systems Thinking and Modeling Workshop; 2006

In the U.S. there is still a major emphasis on the right-hand side of this Figure, about 97 percent of all of the dollars spent on health flows into these right-hand compartments with microscopic emphasis on the left-hand side. Applying systems dynamics should drive policy making to the left-hand side, not abandoning the good work in some of the other areas, but trying to work even harder to keep the population as far to the left side of this graph as much as possible.[100] The reaction of other balancing or reinforcing feedback loops to these actions is the cause of policy resistance or willing follow through observed in the real world as the system attempts to restore equilibrium or transform. From a systems thinking perspective, systems consist of interrelated feedback loops where actions try to alter the balance of the feedback loops.

Similarly, the counter-intuitive results of actions are the result of incomplete understanding of the structure of the feedback loops present in a system.[98] Two types of feedback loops include:

1. Reinforcing (positive) loops and
2. Self-correcting (negative) loops exist.

The former describes situations where a disturbance within the loop's variables is an amplified cause-effect causing exponential growth or decline in the system. The latter is disturbance resisting the system directed toward a state of equilibrium to achieve a goal. Although it is easy to infer the behavior of each of these loops in isolation, if a system includes many interacting feedback loops, as is often the case, it becomes impossible to predict how the system will behave. Since health is complex, it has many inputs and outputs, which operate independently upon one another in multiple overlapping feedback loops. For example, device manufacturers adjust their costs and prices to reimbursement levels, and reimbursement levels are set to prevailing of structures. All dynamics observed in systems are derived from shifts in feedback loop dominance as a system evolves over time.[25,86] In this context, actions can be interpreted as influences attempting to shift the balance of power among the system's feedback loops. The actual behavior of the system depends on which loop is stronger, the positive or the negative.[2] For example, preventive diabetes services, such as nutrition education are not compensated. This policy drives more expensive services such as emergency treatment of diabetic shock and amputations.

In the figures above, standard epidemiological approaches or fixation on curative care or insurance coverage addresses one issue at a time. A systems dynamics approach extends linear analyses by placing reinforcing and balancing loops into perspective. Rather than focus on one stock and flow, defining the community with this frame of reference facilitates identification of systemic patterns and behaviors among the entire system at large. The goal is to decrease contributing factors to the burden of disease. In the US, there is less investment in social services when compared to other countries. In virtually all societies, the heaviest burden of illness falls upon those who are economically and socially marginalized, disenfranchised, or oppressed. These members are more vulnerable to disease outbreaks and unhealthy habits contributing to poor health and reinforce each other as a vicious cycle of unhealthy balancing loops. A systems dynamics and systems thinking approach challenges leaders to identify conditions to create and sustain health. For these reasons, systems dynamics models provide a more precise and accurate framework for understanding and preventing the conditions that perpetuate health disparities.[100]

Time Delays in Feedback Loops

Typically, an action follows its trigger. However, causes and effects are often not close in time and space.[98,103,104] These **delays** make systems more complex. In fact, they slow the learning process by reducing the ability to accumulate experience, test hypotheses, and apply findings. This behavior inhibits an ability intervene to improve a particular situation.[98] For example, as more regulations are created to control the behavior of a complex system, the more the system may deviate from the desired outcome.[105] Commenting on the complexity of the Australian health care system, Sturmberg et al.[106] wrote the prevailing trends to use disease protocols, economic levers, and stovepipe programs to manage the health system are flawed ultimately leading to unintended consequences.

Further, if consequences of actions are not apparent, agents will take measures to make systems converge to the desired end state without giving it time to absorb the effects of the actions and respond adequately. For example, a component of 21st Century Cures included the Helping Families in Mental Health Crisis Act of 2016. This was a landmark "regulatory relief" mental health reform policy. The bill was designed to increase the availability of psychiatric hospital beds and boost treatment for young mental health patients as the most significant attempt at mental health reform in decades.[107] As illustrated in the figure below typical expectations of decision-making is characterized in the single-Decision Open Loop View. In reality, as shown by the Feedback View, the result is **delaying or oscillating behavior** in which systems overshoot or lags behind equilibrium.

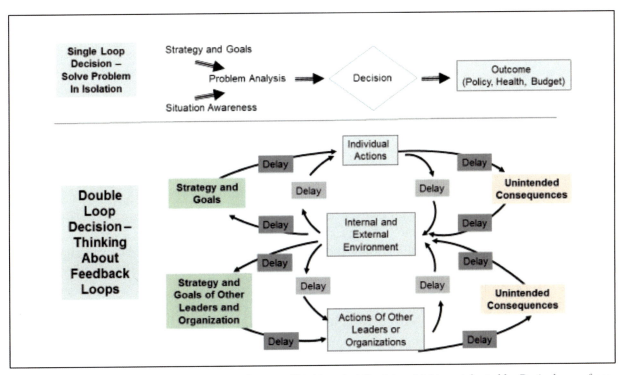

Part 2, Chapter 8, Figure 16: Linear Versus Systems Thinking And Decision-Making. Adapted by D. Anderson from Milstein, B, Overview of Systems Dynamics Simulation Modeling, Systems Thinking and Modeling Workshop; 2006

This behavior becomes more prominent where some delays are "unobservable": A context in which effective decision-making based on intuition or experience becomes elusive.[103,104] For example, pay-for-performance payment models aim to improve the quality of care at lower cost and better health may encourage aggressive treatment without concern for life expectancy or adverse effects. Contrary to expectation, these models have had no effect on mortality[108] or Medicare spending.[109] Similarly, clinical practice guidelines designed to improve the quality of care and reduce variations have not reduced socioeconomic disparities in the treatment of diabetes[110] and could increase the education costs of patients with multiple chronic conditions.[111]

Non-Linear Relationships

This source of dynamic complexity means the response (effect) of the system to an action (cause) is not always linearly proportional. Non-linear relationships enable triggered steps to cause a shift in dominance from one loop to another. This action exacerbates the frequency of changes among the system's feedback loops resulting in dynamic complexity. The same actions may trigger unpredictable consequences because the response of the system is based on the balancing loop power among its feedback loops. The presence of these relations increases complexity because the system's response to a disturbance will be different and will depend on the current state. The present fee-for-service reimbursement system discourages sharing of responsibility for patient care between organizations by limiting payment to only one service at a time or in isolation. Failure to recognize this property is one of the problems with the health system where stovepipes of care with minimal attention to patient handoff, communication, and continuity. Key to the success of a complex system is observing nonlinear interactions of the components.[112]

Effect of Dynamic Complexity on Decision-Making

High levels of dynamics affect human decision-making. Often decisions do not generate optimal or even reasonable outcomes. There are many reasons for under-performance in complex situations. Two reasons are of vital importance.

First, the principle of "bounded rationality" developed by Nobel Laureate, Herbert Simon, states humans suffer from two bounds of rationality. The first is due to limited information processing capabilities. When humans are faced with complexity, they focus on reduced amounts of information and simplify their mental cause-effect maps by using linear thinking while ignoring the side effects of their decisions. Their mental models are flawed. The second aspect of bounded rationality is due to the cognitive skills and memory limitations. Even with perfect information about the cause-effect maps, humans are unable to work out the consequences of their actions. In such situations, only a formal modeling approach can act as a learning catalyst and improve the decision-making performance. Only formal modeling can serve as a learning mediator to improve the decision-making performance. Therefore, their mental models are not an accurate representation of the real world. And these different bounds of rationality must be overcome for effective double loop learning to occur."[102]

Second, the misperception of feedback drives differing responses. The principle of "bounded rationality" applies in all types of decision-making. However, its effect is amplified in dynamic situations. It has been observed humans perform poorly, about their potential, in cases involving dynamic complexity. Experiments have shown the performance of humans decreased dramatically in the presence of high levels of dynamic complexity. This behavior is truer when subjects have considerable experience or when incentives have been given as a reward. These situations are used as evidence to prove the validity of the "misperception of feedback" hypothesis, which suggests mental models are deficient. Humans ignore feedback, do not appreciate time delays between actions and consequences, and are insensitive to the non-linearity's between a system's elements evolving over time.[49]

System Dynamics in Action

System Dynamics (SD), developed in the late 1950s at the Massachusetts Institute of Technology's (MIT) Sloan School of Management by Jay Forrester tried to apply the principles of feedback, control, and management to social systems dynamics. The basis of System Dynamics is the behavior of a system is caused by internal structures. SD assumes system structures are composed of feedback loops in which delays and nonlinearities drive a system's behavior. SD aims to model and predict responses of complex systems to decisions so their leverage points can be identified or their structures are redesigned to eliminate undesirable behavior. The SD intervention process is further divided into three phases.[97]

First, any SD model should have a purpose and a defined problem or undesirable behavior. The variables of interest are described as a model and graphical representation of their behavior over time. The factors believed to cause the behavior are identified, and the relationships between them described and modeled in the form of causal loop diagrams (CLDs). The relationship between the causal structures and observed behavior referred to as a dynamic hypothesis: an initial explanation of how a system's structure is causing the observed behavior. A parallel description of the decision-making process is conducted to determine how agents in the system transform information into decisions to include the information flows in the CLDs. This phase is essentially the conceptual, qualitative phase of the intervention. It is important to emphasize this phase should not be conducted by SD experts alone. Involving those who are part of the systems or in problematic situations early on help "capture" better mental models with first-hand knowledge about the causes of the problem.[113]

Second, the model building must be carefully developed as a qualitative structure describing the problem and summarized using CLDs. Next is a computer-based behavioral model to reflect the qualitative structure to illustrate stocks and flows as variables. The stocks (subject to accumulation and depletion processes over time) and the flows (determine the time-related movement of units from a stock to another or location) are determined. The relationships between the stocks and flows are defined. A link is established between the variables and the dynamic behaviors. The quantitative nature of this phase makes it the most important one regarding generating insights about the situation. Many software programs have been written for SD modeling to make the process easy and accessible to individuals even without strong computational background.

Finally, testing and use of the model in the problem situation is required. Before the model is used for policy analysis, it is necessary to build confidence or validity of the model. Because a model replicates reality, replication at a satisfactory level such as the time path of stocks and flows in a system improves decision-making.[87,97] Once a model is validated, it can be used for different purposes such as testing the impact of different health market policies or single payer systems, exploring what-if scenarios such as disease outbreaks, or optimizing some sub-structures in the system such as Medicaid expansion. Ultimately, the model is used as a base to derive policies or structural changes.

System Dynamics Modeling For Health Systems

Health systems are complex. This may explain the disappointing results of current policies attempting to improve the performance of health systems. From an SD perspective, health systems exhibit high levels of dynamic complexity and are subject to counter-intuitive behavior and policy resistance. Although a small fraction of a governments' budget is allocated to health, results have not matched expectations. In this context, SD modeling can be an effective tool to address the concerns and contribute towards improved health system performance. The contribution of SD modeling methods can deal effectively with strategic and tactical problems involving aggregate flows of patients and resources.[114]

SD modeling offers unique opportunities to improve a decision-makers' understanding of the sources of their systems' under-performance. For example, since SD uses both qualitative and quantitative tools, analyses lead to consensus building, better understanding, information sharing, and cross organization boundary learning. Before describing the possibilities of SD modeling in health systems and health care management policy, it is necessary to explore the reasons make health systems highly dynamic and complex.

First, health systems involve many interacting feedback loops. These loops occur as the health system elements interact and have a mutual influence on each other. These interactions cannot be adequately captured by linear models as they are inherently a straight chain of cause and effect relationships. For example, to facilitate collaborative design of an improved stroke care unit, a system dynamics (SD) model was used in the early stages of planning. The figure below illustrates the results of a six-part workshop. CLDs were created by a multi-professional team to illustrate how SD and CLDs facilitated an explicit description of patient-centered stroke care processes.

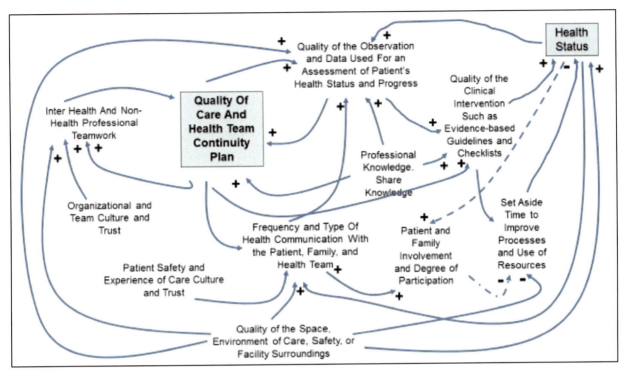

Part 2, Chapter 8, Figure 17: Illustration on How Causal Loop Diagrams Are Used For Mapping Stroke Care Processes. Adapted by D. Anderson from Elf M, Putilova, Mariya, von Koch, Lena, Öhrn, Kerstin. Using System Dynamics for Collaborative Design: A Case Study. BMC Health Services Research. 2007;7:123

The method supported the conceptualization of stroke care by discussions of the care key variables and processes. This approach contributed to a dialogue and common understanding of frictions and inefficiencies in the delivery of care. Moreover, the opportunity to experiment with a model to support the significance of the dependent and independent variables in a visual manner and develop sustainable solutions related to a patient's health contributes to higher reliability.[115]

From this example, the presence of interrelated feedback loops makes the design of sound policies less complicated than it appears. A well-designed action to improve flow and hands-on care was illustrated using negative to the positive feedback loops. These loops illustrated the instability and unpredictability of care process and outcomes. From this example, leaders can observe health systems involve feedback structures, which make them highly dynamic and complex. The use of SD modeling is of paramount importance if improved performance of health systems at any level is to be achieved.

Second, health systems decisions involve many delays at all levels. This means cause and effect in these systems are not close in time and space. For example, there is a delay between the time a doctor is needed and the time at when the doctor is fully trained and available--a gap in the supply and demand. This situation renders management of such cases problematic because if consequences of actions are not immediately visible, decision makers tend to take dysfunctional actions while trying to restore the system to a desirable state. Similarly, all too often there is a delay between the appearance of symptoms and access to care. For instance, in a cohort study, patients with *Chlamydia* did not seek treatment once symptoms appeared but delayed consulting a doctor until infertility became apparent and treatment was no longer effective.[116] Understanding delays and dealing with their consequences is a challenge if they are coupled with strongly interconnected feedback loops. The remedy is to adopt a formal modeling approach such as SD for better problem representation and analysis.

Third, health care systems involve many non-linear relationships. This relation means a response to an input (action) in a system may be different because the reply will depend on the system's conditions. As the global population ages, immense pressures on hospitals and other health services are compromising their abilities to meet the growing demand. SD modeling and simulation can be used to counter this increasing pressure. For example, policy analysts studied the effects acute bed blockage problems in the Irish health system. The current demand-supply gaps result in prolonged waiting times in emergency departments (EDs). However, overcrowding in EDs stems from the delayed patient flows to inpatient wards congested with inpatients waiting for beds in post-acute facilities. Bed blocking in acute hospitals caused substantial cost burdens. A system dynamics model assessed the flow of elderly patients to gaining a better understanding of the complexity created by the system's parameters.[117]

The model evaluated the stocks and flows that are typical and proposed interventions to overcome delayed discharges, increased costs, and anticipated growth of the elderly population. For example, if patients waited for a long time before admission, the treatment time was considerably longer as the patient's health situation worsened while waiting for treatment, preventing other admissions, and lengthening waiting times for patients on the wait list. If shorter lengths of stays are allocated to particular patients, the probability of relapse after treatment has increased. This delay may lead to subsequent admission, the occupation of more beds, and lengthening of the waiting list. The presence of non-linear relationships make it difficult to accurately predict the behavior of a health system and complicates management decision-making. Also, in this case, policy makers used the model to identify risks arising from the unintended consequences of new policies designed to overcome flaw policies or process associated with the delayed discharge of elderly patients.[117]

Finally, health systems involve "hard" and "soft" elements. Health organizations are beginning to embrace the sciences of safety, improvement, human factors, and complexity to transform their organizations into a culture of high reliability. For example, analyzing variables such as health team motivation, fatigue, responses to incentives, psychological safety could result in healthier outcomes and high reliable patient care. Making decisions on "hard" variables is not difficult. The data and information are available, understood, and not subject to much argument.

However, health systems involve a strong human element and the "soft" variables, represent aspects of human behavior and responses must be taken into account. For example, nurses are the front lines of patient safety and quality processes. Nurses are required to understand and develop the skills needed to improve these care processes and continuously improve processes. These changes demand nurses understand the complex demands of providing harm-free care and system dynamics to create the conditions for improved outcomes, health organization performance, interprofessional development, and teamwork. SD has the potential to create safer patient care environments and mitigates unsafe safe nursing care into at-risk and unsafe nursing care. Since the variables complicate problem analysis as they are not easily quantifiable and their effects are not subject to rapid consensus SD methods can easily accommodate such variables and allow more realistic analysis of health systems.[118]

Reflection

This chapter and its' examples illustrate how health systems are dynamic and complex and why SD is an appropriate method to be applied. The complexity of increasing the health of a community must be approached systematically. Health systems face increasing demands and reduced resources. An equitable approach to improving health system sustainability including societal needs, financial constraints, and intensifying environmental expectations is required. Growing attention to sustainability in health services delivery or public health services and finding solutions among community health and non-health actors and stakeholders is intensifying.

However, technical adequacy and elegance of SD are not the reasons to adopt SD modeling. The methods offer many advantages over the "hard" modeling techniques. The benefits include the ability to involve the different stakeholders in the modeling process and more interaction with those involved in developing policies and strategies. Adoption results in sharing of knowledge, an opportunity for questioning assumptions in a non-threatening environment, enhancement of group learning, and easier convergence to sustainable solutions for complex problems.[98] For these reasons, SD should become a widely used technique in health settings.

Chapter 9: Uncovering Archetypes to Prevent Dysfunction

Introflection

Systems archetypes first studied in the 1960s and 1970s by Jay Forrester, Donella Meadows, Gene Bellinger, were summarized in the seminal 1990 book, *The Fifth Discipline: The Art and Practice of the Learning Organization*, Peter Senge created common archetypes or mental concepts as the most common set of patterns of behavior in organizations. The word archetype refers to the original pattern or model from which all things of the same kind are copied or on which they are based. When applied to systems or cultures, archetypes have a tendency of reoccurring regardless of setting and constantly seek expression. Some archetypes are highly desirable, such as the archetype of *mother*, while others are not, such as the archetype of *monster*. Sadly, they can both co-exist and thus lead to pathology, i.e. *monster mother*. The US health system, especially health insurance markets are showing symptoms of increasing instability and many pathologies. Various players perceive they are doing so poorly they attempt to change the strategy only to find out the fix failed and a problem emerged elsewhere. These micro actions include health care teams who opt out of the insurance payment system, set up "concierge" practices, or open urgent-care centers. Patients now choose foreign countries for care, buy pharmaceuticals over the Internet, or opt out of the medical system entirely because they cannot afford it. Health systems like Geisinger who are setting up their insurance system, hiring physicians as employees, bundling payment systems between providers, and giving patient satisfaction guarantees. Key players such as pharmaceutical companies, health plans, and device manufacturers, show little interest in the main new strategies. These actions are characteristic of the typical archetypes as described by Senge.

Systems archetypes – mental models are common and usually represent reoccurring patterns of behavior or outcomes, both negative and positive. Unless uncovered earlier rather than later, these patterns may result in unintended consequences or frustration and spread to other parts of the system. Dysfunctional systems archetypes – as a policy, organization, and leadership pathology should provide additional insight into structures, policies, and processes from which negative behavior over time plagues the system. For example, the US spends more on health services than the following countries combined: Japan, Germany, France, China, UK, Italy, Canada, Brazil, Spain, and Australia. The US ranks in the middle or below in health statistics and mortality when compared to 17 other developed nations. Sadly, by many accounts, 30 cents of every dollar spent on medical care in America is wasted, which amounts to $750 billion annually. Much of this waste is attributed to the pharmaceutical industry's perverse practices, prescribing practices, and patient behavior such as lack of adherence.[119,7] In this case, several archetypes should alert health leaders and policy makers to prevent the unintended consequences. Collectively, archetypes should challenge health leaders to consider the merits of seeking out pathologies and organizational dysfunctions and generate sustainable solutions. The key is seeking out and uncovering the archetypes.

Because complex adaptive health systems behave differently than simple non-living systems, it is helpful to understand the common characteristics they possess and the problems they present. Systems thinkers may choose to describe consequential patterns of interaction within health systems as pathologies: waste, inefficient processes of care, poor health outcomes, disparities in health, and preventable deaths. For example, when compared to 7 countries, Americans have the second highest rate of chronic disease, Australia being number one. With the funds, the US spends on healthcare, what's missing? This statistic reflects the poor preventative care and lack of attention to lifestyle habits, such as diet, exercise, stress, and sleep. More American adults and children are becoming insulin-resistant due to junk food based diets, sugar drinks, processed grains, and chemical additives. Insulin dysfunctions place individuals in a state of constant inflammation thus driving up chronic disease rates.[120,7] National policies such as less emphasis on preventive care and healthy lifestyle adoption or "fix me now" cultures reinforce this behavior.

Increasing complexity in a system has its advantages and disadvantages. Compared with simple systems, a highly adaptive complex system is typically able to process more information, anticipate changes more accurately, learn quickly, act more flexibly, and respond more appropriately to a wide range of circumstances.[9] On the other hand, more complexity can mean more problems (and opportunities). Complex systems, especially health systems have more subsystems to organize and maintain. Therefore, there are more opportunities for risk of errors, harm, and death in healthcare settings. Current national level payment policies do not reward or incentivize reliability or better health outcomes. In fact, it can be argued medical errors are the leading cause of death in the US—higher than heart disease, higher than cancer. The errors include inappropriate medical treatment, hospital-acquired infections, unnecessary surgeries, and adverse drug reactions. One in four patients is harmed by preventable mistakes or about 250,000 patients die from medication errors per year.[121,7] Several archetypes-organizational pathologies-are indicators of problems leaders must seek out when working with complex systems. System archetypes can be used as a mental conceptual tool to understand the dynamics of behaviors that have manifested an unwanted condition or pathology.

Recognizing System Archetypes with Circles and Loops

The theory behind systems archetypes is that situations with unwanted results or side effects can be mapped to common behavioral models. These systems can be expressed by circles of causality. Identifying a system archetype and finding leverage points enables dynamic changes in a system to create sustainable solutions and better health outcomes. Uncovering archetypes requires an understanding of the basics.

First, circles of causality characterize most archetypes. The basic idea of system thinking is every action triggers a reaction—positive, negative, neutral--feedback in the form of reinforcing and balancing feedback. The figure below provides a typical visual.

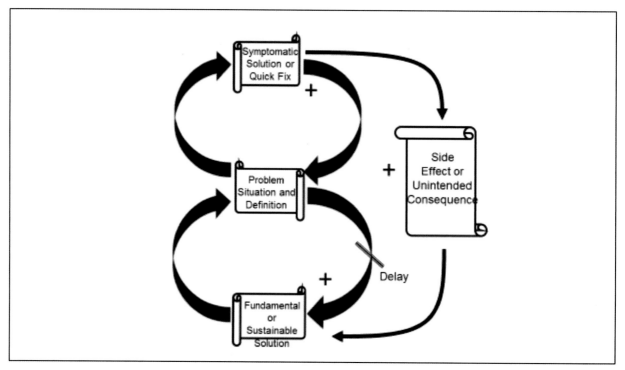

Part 2, Chapter 9, Figure 18: Illustration Of The Typical Archetype And Reinforcing Or Balancing Loops, created by D. Anderson

Sometimes, feedback (or reaction) does not occur immediately; it contains delays. Any system can be drawn as a structure or diagram using circles of causality with actions, feedback, and delays. For example, continuous quality improvement (CQI) has proven to be successful in reducing costs, reducing complications, and improving patient satisfaction. Hospitals and clinics that have embraced a culture of safety and quality improvement have experienced declines in patient mortality, rates of adverse events, costs of care, and delays in diagnosis and treatment. One of the IOM's six specific aims for improvement is timely care – reducing waits and harmful delays in care. Unnecessary transportation of patients causes delay or lack of information transfer. Extra costs are incurred to rework the effects of delays. Defects, corrections, adjustments and inaccurate or incomplete information cause problems associated with lack of feedback and delays. A misapplied, illegible or improperly labeled blood tube can cause errors or delays in processing. In fact, according to the literature and national data, the most frequent claims in the ambulatory care setting stem from missed and delayed diagnoses.[122]

Second, as part of the circles of causality reinforcing feedback (+) loops are prevalent. Reinforcing feedback (or amplifying feedback)--Vicious (Harmful) or Virtuous (Helpful) -- accelerates the given trend of a process. If the trend line is ascending, the reinforcing (positive) feedback will speed up the growth. If the trend line is descending, it will accelerate the decline. Actions magnify future problems such as lack of trust, delegation, and empowerment. For example, as the supervisor's supportive behavior increases, employee performance related to the quality of care and personal attention to patients increases which reinforce supervisor's supportive behavior, which in turn reinforces employee behavior – virtuous reinforcing loop. However, when a supervisor's supportive behavior diminishes, or attention gets diverted, employee performance declines, driving worsening supervisor support which further decreases performance – a vicious reinforcing loop. Worse, as the quality of care provided increases, research shows the utilization of services will increase, driving increased workload. Since there is no compensating increase in staff coverage, the increased workload ultimately drives down staff motivation, which drives down the level of respectful care given, and ultimately diminishes the quality of care provided. This cycle of human activity is typical of a balancing loop – despite the change in the quality of care. Utilization of more staff time is limited because of change or policy resistance demonstrated by staff behavior. Without an increase in staffing, this will continue as a balancing feedback loop.

Third, depending on the problem balancing feedback (−) loops will be present or emerge from somewhere. Balancing or stabilizing feedback works if a goal exists. Balancing process intends to reduce a gap between a current state and the desired state such as access to care. The balancing (negative) feedback adjusts to the current status (i.e., delayed or extended wait times for care) to a desirable target (i.e., standards for access to care) regardless whether the trend line is descending or ascending. To illustrate, a study of access to care by the Veteran's Affairs (VA) to veteran's health facilitates measured the relationship between waiting times for health care services and mortality. Analysis of available appointments—circles of causality and increased morbidity and deaths--feedback at 89 Veterans Affairs (VA) indicated Veterans who visited a VA medical center with facility-level wait times of 31 days or more had significantly higher odds of mortality—viscous feedback loop. The association between long wait times for outpatient health care created negative health outcomes. Variation in access, resources, and the results was notable across VA medical centers. Actions should focus on the causes of long waits for health care and development of effective resource allocation policies –balancing loop feedback to decrease long waits for health care services.[123] This study illustrates the forces of limiting growth and an inability to achieve equilibrium. Balancing loops reduce the impact of change.

Finally, as part of the feedback loops delays can be expected. Delays in systems and policy implementation can cause individuals to perceive a response to an action incorrectly. For example, there are long lead times—a large lead-lag or stock-and-flow problem—between action and effect, especially in primary care preventative medicine. These long times cause an under or overestimation of the needed action and results creating oscillation, instability or even breakdown. Unintended consequences will occur. In addition to the long delays in cause and effect, many leaders believe good intentions and logic are sufficient to achieve outcomes. There is no obligation among either leaders or legislators/regulators to produce—in advance of action—evidence-of-desired-effects.[124] For example, current health system reform efforts recognize success requires a shift from fragmented coordination of care from highly specialized care to primary care and prevention. The national patient-centered medical home (PCMH) model demonstration represents an innovative model to integrate primary care services into specialty care, reimbursement reform, new information technology, and the chronic care model. The primary outcomes are promising, however quantitative assessments –creating oscillations–have not been conducted. The expectation of short-term cost savings such as decreased inpatient, specialty care, and ancillary services utilization may be unrealistic. An investment in information infrastructure and training practices to mitigate instability and delay might be needed.. Interpretation and expectations must be tempered. It takes four to five years –delay– to yield noticeable results yet many organizations are under pressure to report results in less than two years, some shorter. Analysts should not jump to conclusions about the feasibility of PCMH.

Refresher on Senge's Archetypes to Identify Systems Pathologies

Given the knowledge about systems archetypes, problem-solvers can apply the principles and arrive at sustainable solutions and prevent long-term or delayed unintended consequences. The systems archetypes knowledge provides guidelines for determining what archetype is at play and how to apply the intervention to increase the success of an intended consequence such as better health for a population or increased quality of life and productivity for a community. For example, charging customers co-pays has the expected consequence of reducing casual over-utilization, recreational surgeries, and whine-on-demand hypochondriacally office visits. If systems go unchecked, the actual consequence leads to the elimination of minor utilization including preventive checkups, pap smears, and mammograms. Later this could increase major utilization for the big things checkups did not catch or cause some individuals to forego the necessary treatment (chemotherapy, cardiac catheterization) and simply die rather than impoverish their families. A summary of the most common systems archetypes is summarized below. They explained in more detail along with special forms:

- Shifting the Burden: a symptom is solved with short-term and basic solutions. The solution produces side effects affecting the basic solution. The attention then shifts to the short-term solution or the side effects.
- Fixes that Fail or Back Fire: the solution is rapidly implemented to address the symptoms of an urgent problem. This quick fix sets in motion unintended consequences not evident at first but end up adding to the symptoms.
- Limits to Growth or Success: A given effort initially generates positive performance. However, over time the effort reaches a constraint that slows down the overall performance no matter how much energy is applied.
- Drifting or Eroding Goals: As a gap between goal and actual performance is realized, the conscious decision is to lower the target. The effect is a gradual decline in system performance.
- Growth and Underinvestment: Growth approaches a limit avoidable with investments in a capability or a service capacity. However, a decision to not invest in performance drives degradation further resulting in a demand not to invest.
- Success to the Successful: Two or more efforts compete for the same finite resources. The more successful effort gets a disproportionately larger allocation of the resources to the detriment of the others.
- Escalation: parties take mutually threatening actions which escalate their retaliation attempting to "one-up" each other.
- The Tragedy of the Commons: Multiple entities enjoy the benefits of a common resource but do not pay attention to the effects of using the common resource. Eventually, the resource dwindles, and the activities of all entities in the system perish.

Understanding and Uncovering Archetypes in the Context of Health

By facilitating an understanding of systems archetypes: including concepts, preventive actions, and health leadership imperatives as a storyline, a mental image can be created. Thinking about the archetypes using circles and feedback loops can be extremely helpful at any level. Circles of causality and feedback loops can be used to analyze variations in supply and demand for health care services between individual and community health. Typically called 'neighborhood effects' or 'place effects,' these phenomena capture how a person's environment affect their health in both the short term and the long term.[125]

These storylines are universal and can be applied to the understanding of emerging manifestations or pathologies inside organizations or at the policy levels. For example, controlling costs and utilization may become a success, and the success becomes accentuated with more attempts to control costs without regard to quality of care or patient behaviors and attitudes toward personal health. In another example, studies on provider practice and variation capture the heterogeneity in provider behavior and how health team practices become reinforced within peer networks. These analyses have uncovered practices inconsistent with state-of-the-art evidence-based medicine, which resulted in the provision of ineffective care.[126]

Systems archetypes have a structure, pattern, and behavior. To further illustrate, the figure above illustrates a structure is comprised of variables and feedback loops—one or more, of which, contain a delay. In health, feedback loops are used to describe 'vicious circles such as between lower socioeconomic status and ill health or malnutrition. The structure of systems archetypes is typically depicted through causal loop diagrams, a tool from system dynamics. The picture shows the typical conceptual structure of the "fixes that fail" archetype. These structures have variables: symptom, quick fix, and unintended consequence. The flow between the fix and unforeseen consequence contains delay or reason for the archetype. Two feedback loops are present in this structure: balancing loop for a quick fix and a detrimental reinforcing loop for the pathological manifestation of the unintended consequence. For example, controlling the length of stay and other in-patient cost structures drives drive-through surgeries until those come under control too. Alternatively, they try to control pharmaceutical costs by refusing to reimburse for over-the-counter drugs, and suddenly there is a version of Elixir, the same drug just twice as strong so reimbursed can be pursued. This behavior is the adaptive part of a complex adaptive system. The system perceives proscriptive regulation as damage and routes around it.

This action usually contributes to unintended consequences of the behavioral pattern. Variables are those that form part of the feedback loops to modify and are modified by other variables. For example, limits to success, growth, and underinvestment, and tragedy of the commons contain variables acting as external constraints to these systems. For example, the "systems that fail" archetype has the "squeaky wheel" as its storyline. In this archetype, a quick fix is applied to a "squeaky wheel") to reduce its symptom and "noise" associated with it. The storyline gets complicated when unintended effects or variables of the quick fix become consequential. These effects start to add to the problem symptoms making the quick fix less or totally ineffective. The systems archetypes profiled in the following pages are well worth pondering:

Archetype -- Shifting the Burden

Concept: Shifting the Burden illustrates the tension between the attraction (and relative ease and low cost) of devising symptomatic solutions to obvious problems and the long-term impact of fundamentally sustainable solutions aimed at underlying structures producing the pattern of behavior in the first place. Access to health services along with free insurance shifts the responsibility of personal health-to-health teams rather than an individual practice of a healthy lifestyle. The tension between the two is understandable. For example, the government attempts to solve social problems with entitlement but fosters more dependency since the word "entitlement" signals recipients feel they have the right to something. Sometimes, entitlement recipients do not know where the money comes from and warns the government to leave Medicare alone. Long-term solutions demand deeper understanding about underlying problems. Long-term solutions take a long time to formulate, require a relatively large commitment of funds and time, and test a leaders' patience in the face of pressures for quick fixes. The diet fad industry encourages individuals to find quick-fix solutions rather than live sustainable, healthy lifestyles with exercise and proper nutrition.

Preventive Actions: Focus on the basic solution. Apply quick solutions to the symptom to gain time while working on a long-term solution. Explore potential side-effects of any proposed solution. Identify the initial problem symptom. Map all "quick fixes" appearing to be keeping the problem under control. Determine the impact of the symptomatic solutions on other parts of the system. Identify fundamental solutions. Develop multiple perspectives. Find interconnections to fundamental loops and links between the interactions and the fundamental solution causing resistance. Identify high-leverage actions from both perspectives.

Health Leadership's Imperatives: Shifting the Burden is an example of creative tension. Policy resistance or overcoming resistance to change is a reaction to limits to growth and shifting the burden. When actors attempt to pull a system in a certain direction such as government mandated health insurance benefits the results can be policy resistance. Any new policy, especially if it is defective, just pulls the system producing additional resistance with a result no one likes, but everyone expends considerable effort in maintaining. The way out is to bring in all the actors and use the energy formerly expended on resistance to seeking out mutually satisfactory ways for all goals to be realized — or redefinitions of larger and more important goals everyone can pull toward together. Leaders must seek first to understand, develop patience, and seek deeper connections to the tensions, and then respond. This approach illustrates the challenge of engaging in strategic health leadership in the face of mounting pressure to fix it now (e.g. health insurance schemes). Without a clear and convincing picture of a shared vision such as improved population health, community health and quality of life, the pressure to go for the quick fix may overwhelm the health leader, condemning her/him to a recurring pattern of interventions solving the same problem symptoms associated with today's health system.

Archetype -- Addiction – Special Form of Shifting the Burden

Concept: Addictions are compulsive behavior patterns individuals or organizations unconsciously do to bring temporary relief. At the individual level, individuals misperceive addictions as actions to solve real needs or satisfy sufferings. As a result, individuals grasp for alcohol, gambling, hedonic experiences, romantic love, self-improvement programs, peer approval, new possessions, and all sorts of gratifications to escape deeper problems. For example, medication and opioid addiction is a major individual and national issue. Unintended addition or feeling better through the use of drugs (dependency is the unintended side-effect). Taking pain relievers to address chronic pain rather than visiting a doctor to address the underlying problem is a form of shifting the burden.

The Addiction archetype does not just happen to individuals, but can be built into larger systems – agriculture addicted to subsidies, nurses addicted to unions and the banking sector addicted to bailouts. Interveners such as policymakers with good intentions want to solve problems and remove the burden from individuals within a system. Unfortunately, these individuals do not learn how to deal with the problem themselves. Then, gridlock appears. For example, gridlock on how to solve the medication and opioid addiction crises arises with implementation government programs designed to increase the recipient's dependency on the government or a health organization versus a preventive care and health promotion strategy thus shifting the burden to the government rather than the individual. This action is a solution to a systemic problem reducing or disguising the symptoms but does nothing to solve the underlying problem. Eventually, the system deteriorates; more and more of the solution is then required. The system becomes more and more dependent on the intervention and less and less able to maintain the desired state. Rather than find long-term solutions, they pursue quick fixes to relieve symptoms under the auspice of true problem solving. The addicted, are now tied to the helper for success; are less capable, responsible, and willing to solve its problems in the future.

Preventive Actions: The archetype provides a starting point for breaking gridlock by identifying chains of problem symptoms and solutions between functions, departments, or organizations. The best way out of this trap is to avoid getting in. Beware of symptom – relieving or signal – denying policies or practices not addressing the problem. Take the focus off short-term relief and invest in long-term prevention efforts.

Health Leadership's Imperatives: As the intervener, work to restore or enhance the system's ability to solve its problems. If individuals have an unstoppable dependency, build the system's capabilities back up for removing the intervention. Do it right away. Some view Shifting the Burden as necessary in certain cases of desperation to ward off suffering or kick the can down the road. Since Shifting the Burden does not solve the cause, the same problems will reappear. The health leader will need to continue spending time and resources to prop up the system.

Archetype -- Fixes That Fail or Back Fire

Concept: When Leaders say, "I thought this ____ was fixed? Why is it worse? The Fixes that Fail archetype is at work. This archetype is also a reflection of the perils of reductionist and linear thinking. Despite their best intentions leaders find themselves dealing with the same symptoms over and over again. When problem symptoms are assumed to be unique circumstances in their isolated stovepipe unconnected to other parts of the larger whole system, one assumes a reasonable response and will be effective. Fixes That Fail is similar to Shifting the Burden. A health leader's response is aimed at the problem symptom rather than spending time on the more challenging and time-consuming task of identifying the underlying, systemic problem (or as is more often the case, the system of challenges). The difference is the unintended consequence emerges from the quick-fix. It functions as a reinforcing loop, exacerbating the initial problem symptom. By contrast, Shifting the Burden suggests a problem has not been addressed only shifted for a limited time. Fixes That Fail display steadily eroding scenarios, where initial problem symptoms are compounded by the Band-Aid fix. The reinforcing loop contains a delay and contributes to a deteriorating problem symptom, not despite the fix but because of it.

Preventive Actions: Focus on removing the fundamental cause of the symptom. If a temporary, a short-term solution is needed; develop a two-tier approach of simultaneously applying the fix and planning out a long-term solution. Use the archetype to connect all side-effects of any intervention. For example, rules to govern a system can lead to rule beating — perverse behavior appears as obeying the process or procedure. The solution is to design or redesign processes or rules to release creativity; not a means to work on the process or procedure. Focus on the predetermined direction of achieving the purpose of the process or procedure. The 2016 Cures Act advances regulatory science. The act was designed to speed discovery, development, and delivery of medical products to prevent or cure disease and improve health while applying evidence-based guidelines to assure the safety and effectiveness of medical products.[8]

Health Leadership's Imperatives: Use scenarios to brainstorm for root causes, unintended consequences, high-leverage decision points, and possible side-effects. Solving a problem tends to create more problems. The key to Fixes That Fail is isolating delays in the loops. This situation makes the connection between the fix and the deteriorating problem symptoms hard to identify. Uncovering root causes requires commitment, setting aside biases, and patience to find sustainable long-term solutions.

Archetype -- Limits to Growth or Success

Concept: Expect resistance. Most of the time, unrestricted positive reinforcing behaviors are not possible. There are always limits to growth and movement. The reinforcing process of accelerating expansion will run into a balancing process as the system's boundary is approached. Diminishing returns will be encountered. Efforts to grow are successful initially. However, as the limits are approached, growth tends to lose momentum and begins to flatten. In the end, despite pressure from the growth process, the speed of growth stops and reverses. This archetype shows success can be dangerous to long-term growth as being unsuccessful. By analyzing the growth processes and danger points, leaders can anticipate future problems and eliminate them before they surface as a threat.

Preventive Actions: Focus on removing the limit (or weakening its effect) rather than continuing to drive the reinforcing process of growth. Use the archetype to identify possible balancing processes before they begin to affect growth. Identify links between the growth processes and limiting factors to determine ways to manage the balance between the two. Other preventive actions include identification of the growth sources, inherent limits and balancing loops, and determining changes required to deal effectively with the limits. Assess the time needed to change. Is there a discrepancy between the doubling time and the changes needed to support growth? Balance the growth. Identify strategies for achieving system balance. Reevaluate the growth strategy.

Health Leadership's Imperatives: Leaders are encouraged to be "action oriented" and "proactive," constantly engaged in connecting part of the process leading to sustainable solutions or outcomes. Continuously challenge assumptions. Leaders must focus beyond their sphere of influence; they need to examine what is pushing back against their efforts constantly. The counter-force may come from either part of the organization not under the health leader's control or from the external environment. Critical thinking is a key competency for locating and focusing attention on limits to growth. Leaders may find opportunities to either continue the improvement curve or identify counter-force elements in the system and devise new improvement initiatives leading to the removal of the limits.

Archetype -- Attractiveness Principle – Special Form of Limits to Growth

Concept: The archetype takes its name from the dilemma of deciding which of the limits to address first, which is more attractive regarding the future benefit to the desired results are pushed by the effort (or growing action). With limited resources, leaders are faced with comparing the potential future value of removing or reducing slowing measures and any synergies associated with the change. In some cases, the health leader may have few options. The lessons from the Attractiveness Principle, on planning, are similar to Limits to Growth. The archetype is beneficial when addressing how long-term decisions affect the availability of resources, their conversion to key capabilities, and maturation of selected capabilities into core competencies. This approach is the case in when organizations pursue resource-based strategies. These firms face the challenge of constant reinvention if they want a competitive advantage.

Preventive Actions: Focus on identifying interconnected and interdependent limits. Use the archetype to identify potential synergistic tactics to remove the balancing processes before they begin to affect growth. Establish priorities; carefully match available resources with specific slowing actions. Identify the growth engines. Map the growth engine to each limiting or slowing action; establish a time line for each slowing action (avoid fixes before they are required). Map the interdependencies between the slowing actions. Model the dynamics of potential synergies between the slowing actions. Review available resources; develop a list of options. Establish metrics to assess the impact of efforts to reduce or remove slowing actions; periodically reassess slowing actions. Reevaluate plans, expected continuous improvement programs and strategies for potential slowing actions and continuously challenge assumptions.

Health Leadership's Imperatives: The Attractiveness Principle pits leaders against growing complexity, and the interactions between parts are difficult to predict. Although implied in several archetypes, it makes a strong case for dynamic modeling to reveal if synergies emerge from a response to growth engines as the complexity increases.

Archetype -- Drifting or Eroding Goals

Concept: Eroding Goals share similarities with Shifting the Burden - the dynamic tension between a symptomatic solution and a fundamental one. In Eroding Goals, leaders are faced with the performance that fails to meet a goal. They seek a rationale (the symptomatic solution) for changing the goal to one appearing to be more attainable rather than determining what prevents the organization from performing as expected. While coverage under the ACA has increased to some degree, one of the reasons Americans' health care is so poorly managed is they are least likely to have primary care providers. There are 0.5 general physicians per 1,000 individuals in the US, but the average among OECD nations is 1.23.[3] Most Americans state their health team is unfamiliar with their medical history which impacts the quality of care and continuity.[7] Unlike other archetypes, Eroding Goals examines dynamic behaviors in the present is the result of forecasts of the future made in the past. The argument for adjusting the aim is not without merit. The future cannot be known, and forecast turns out to be wrong, there is no harm in making adjustments. Two other forms of Drifting or Eroding goals are worth mentioning.

A form of Eroding Goals -- Drift to Low Performance -- Allows performance to be influenced by past performance. This perception sets up a reinforcing feedback loop over eroding goals and establishes a system of drifting toward low performance. For example, Americans do have shorter waits for non-elective surgeries, compared with other developed nations. Only four percent wait more than six months, which is considerably less than Canadians (14 percent) or British (15 percent). However, when considering how many Americans lack access to any health care at all, the wait-time advantage disappears.[10] Also, twenty-five percent do not visit a doctor when they are sick due to the cost. Twenty-three percent cannot or do not fill prescriptions. This is worse in America than in any of the other countries. In Canada, only 5 percent skipped care, and in the United Kingdom only 3 percent. If patients become ill or injured, lack of access can be devastating.[7] The way out is to keep performance standards high. Instead of being discouraged by the worst, upward drifting goals!

Seeking The Wrong Goal – another form of eroding goals-is reinforcing A Hoping for B. If the goal is defined badly, if it does not measure what it is supposed to measure, if it does not reflect the welfare of the system, then the system cannot possibly produce a desirable result. Systems, like these, have a tendency to produce exactly and only what individuals ask them to produce. For example, the US tracks what individuals do not want (death and cost) rather than what they desire: life, daily functions, and productivity—quality of life. This type of system behavior is particularly sensitive to the goals of feedback loops. If the goals — the indicators of satisfaction of the rules — are defined inaccurately or incompletely, the system will work to produce a result not intended or wanted.

Archetype -- Drifting or Eroding Goals (Continued)

For example, the cost of Medicare was more than 800% above projection and helped create the impression health care is a Right. The recently implemented ACA has guidelines without protections will create lawsuits over confidentiality issues, either for withholding clinically relevant data or for inappropriate transmission of protected medical information. Intended consequences may or may not happen; unintended consequences always do.[1] The way out is specifying indicators, and goals reflect the real desired health outcomes of the system. Do not confuse effort with results or end up with a system producing effort, not result.

Preventive Actions: Stay focused on the vision. Various pressures can take attention away from the real goals and outcomes. Used as a diagnostic tool, it can target drifting performance areas and help organizations attain their visions. Anchor goals to an external benchmark to keep them from sliding. Determine is the drift in performance is the result of conflicts between the stated goal and the implicit aims of the system. Establish a clear transition plan from present reality to the goal, including a realistic time frame for achieving the goal. Identify drifting performance measure. Other preventive actions Look for goals conflicting with the stated goal Identify standard procedures for closing the gap. Examine the goal's history. Has the goal been lowered over time? Clarify a compelling vision to involve everyone and create a clear transition plan.

Health Leader Imperatives: Eroding Goals require critical examination immediate short-term effect and deeper understanding of the gaps, seams, and cause. Leaders typically feel pressure to revise goals to match what the organization is currently capable of achieving. Falling into the trap of Eroding Goals tends to become standard practice, justifiable, and routine. Over time, organizations fall farther and farther behind the expectations. On the other hand, leaders should be asking whether the original goals were specific, measurable, attainable, realistic, time sensitive. Since there are good reasons to adjust goals downward, leaders must take extreme caution when considering an adjustment to goals. The two most important considerations are an honest and rigorous examination of the organization itself and an equally candid look at peers or competitors and their performance, and customer expectations.

With this archetype, Seeking the Wrong Goal, sometimes leaders are aware the goal is only a shortcut. This goal is not in organization's best interests. Leaders set them regardless because they are easy to accomplish, measure, or because someone else set them. Many organizations spend years and pursuing goals and ultimately lead down paths distracting them from reaching their true vision. If surgeons are paid by the number of surgeries performed, then many surgeries will be scheduled. If health teams are given the goal of meeting a lower average time spent with a patient, then the time will decrease. What does this do to the quality of care? The tactic is to be uncompromising and focus energy and resources toward accomplishing a true vision and goal.[11]

Archetype -- Growth and Underinvestment

Concept: The Growth and Underinvestment archetype builds upon Limits to Growth by explicitly addressing a need to invest in its resources, capabilities and core competencies. A growing action seeks to stimulate and reinforce demand while the current performance level may amount to growing action will overcome customers' reluctance to reward the organization with sales. For example, investment in the "curative or sick care system" has not yielded the desired results. Health systems, especially hospitals and medical group practices need to focus on new models of care, payment approaches, and patient engagement strategies have the potential to reshape the delivery system to satisfy the needs of the sickest and vulnerable patients. Several health systems are using community benefit funds to reach beyond the walls of their institutions and address the determinants of health including access to safe housing, healthy food, and employment.[4]

For example, an Affordable Care Act provision requires nonprofit hospitals to perform and publish community health needs assessments. This action may encourage others to follow their lead to shed light on what communities need. These reports, often conducted in partnership with public health agencies and organizations such as the United Way, highlight health inequities—whole neighborhoods lack clean environments, safe streets, good schools, vibrant economies, and other assets to support good health. These partners can put firm numbers on an area's most pressing health problems, such as high rates of obesity, suicide, and substance abuse.[4]

Unique to Growth and Underinvestment is the long-term requirement to continue to keep its capabilities, and core competencies at a level ensure its competitive advantage. There are several characteristics of the investment balancing loops are critical from a health leader's decision-making perspective. First, performance standards may be presented as a constant (no causal influences) but may be subject to the Eroding Goals archetype. This constancy may be situational or may have developed over extended periods of time, as the organization loses confidence in its ability to perform at the level of customer expectations. Second, when coupled with the firm's current performance, performance standards collude to exert a corrosive influence on the perceived investment need. At any given performance standard (regardless of a declining trend it may be exhibiting), if current performance falls short, the adage, "why throw good money after bad" will resonate. Third, as confidence declines, investment declines. Declining performance leads to declining revenue, which reduces cash for investment. Fourth, even if the organization makes an investment, a delay in bringing the increased capacity and capability on line may turn out to be a long run for a short slide.

Preventive Actions: Perceived Need to Invest. Identify related patterns of behavior between capacity investments and performance measures. Shorten the delays between performance declines and when additional capacity is operational. Base investment decisions on external signals, not on standards derived from the past. Identify delays between when performance falls and when additional capacity comes online; minimize acquisition delays and identify shortfalls. Are other parts of the system sluggish from added capacity? Avoid self-fulfilling prophecies.

> **Archetype -- Growth and Underinvestment (Continued)**
>
> Challenge the assumptions to drive capacity investment decisions. Search for different investment inputs. Seek new perspectives on products, services and customer requirements.
>
> <u>Health Leader Imperatives</u>: What Does This Mean? Growth and Underinvestment are the archetypes bringing particular attention to planning for limits. In this case, it is the capabilities, and core competencies give firms a competitive advantage. This approach is part of strategic planning as well as policy formation. It also draws attention to the insidious nature of the failure to meet customer demands over extended periods of time – the constant (albeit hard to notice in any one period) decline in the firm's opinion of itself and its commitment to, and ability to perform at customer demands and expectations.

Archetype -- Success to the Successful

Concept: A common piece of wisdom is not to throw good money after bad. This archetype is associated with the "80/20" rule. The Success to the Successful archetype describes common practices of rewarding good performance with more resources in the expectation performance will continue improving. There is a belief the successful entities have "earned" their fair share of resources with past performance. The downside to this assumption is the continued under-performance of other individuals and departments with no attention or development. At the system level, in the 1990s, managed care was a means to reduce the escalation of health costs. Managed care was based on the concept it was less expensive to prevent ailments than treating them. However, the time lag between Medicare costs cause and effect was forgotten. The focus during the managed care era became next month's budget and abusive denial of care procedures, not patient wellbeing. Short term, linear thinking led to the rationale preventative medicine was too expensive, and most patients change health care plans every 2-3 years. Investing patients with complications such as diabetes, hypertension or smoking was ignored and transferred to the next health plan. Therefore, it was not economically feasible to pay for patient education or in-home screening or smoking cessation programs.[1] Now, the US is paying a high price for delaying and avoiding the value of investing in preventive care.

Preventive Actions: If the winners of the competition are systematically rewarded with the means to win again, a reinforcing feedback loop is created. If it is allowed, the winners eventually take all, while others are marginalized. Policies to level the playing field such as removing some of the advantages of the strongest players or increasing the benefit of the weakest should be pursued. Evaluate the current measurement systems to determine if they are set up to favor established practices over other alternatives. Identify goals or objectives will refocus the definition of success to a broader system. Unfortunately, while the Affordable Care Act tips its hat to prevention, it does nothing to restructure the incentives and ultimately stack up against it. Moreover, as the US population continues to age, the high costs of specialty care will continue to consume the gross national product.

Other preventive actions include investigating historical origins of competencies; identify potential competency traps. Investigate initial conditions and the source of the process or procedures. Evaluate current measurement systems. Are they set up to be fair and balanced? Ask "outsiders" for alternative strategies. Assess effects on the innovative spirit. Is the current system limiting the spirit of experimentation? Teamwork? Are leaders continually scanning the environment for gaps and areas for improvement?

Health Leader Imperatives: Leaders should exercise caution before concluding intrinsic merit is good for performance. This archetype may also reveal what is actually measured. Are the measurements still relevant? Accurate? Have delays caused leaders to reach conclusions that appear to favor one over the others? Take a fresh look at "marginal" performers in a new light. This action may lead to insights to rejuvenate an organization's approach to its internal management.

Archetype -- Tragedy of the Commons

Concept: The Tragedy of the Commons provides unique insights into the effect an unsystemic or fragmented approach to the organizational structure can have on overall, long-term performance. The Commons is set for players, departments, organizations or systems with a shared resource (individuals, materials, space, and tools) made available to multiple organizations. The initial parties for creating the commons are typically economies of scale and convenience. As each person or team claims a share of the Commons, within the context of the goals and objectives and availability of resources over time, the demands on the commons steadily erode toward collapse. For example, many observers cast certain players in the health care arena as villains in the Commons (Health System). After all, they are doing what is rational given the current incentives and rules of the game. The three top participants — providers, payers, patients — do what is in their best interest without concern for cost or efficiency. This behavior is accepted due to current policies but is sending the US health system down a destructive path. Only by eliminating the underlying perverse incentives can the long-term survival of the U.S. health care system be rescue.[6]

For patients, more emphasis must be on responsibility. The current U.S. health system is not structured to provide incentives for preventive care and healthier lifestyle choices. This failure in the Health Commons has led to spiraling costs associated with preventable diseases. By contrast, insurance companies in the Netherlands have devised plans rooted in libertarian paternalism, offering patients discounts for healthy lifestyles and nutritional choices. This approach empowers patients to focus on reducing costs and producing better health. Providers must reconcile the disparity in cost and quality of care for common conditions such as hypertension. A metric for delivering preventive care will encourage health teams to incorporate these procedures into routine practice to make informed decisions. Finally, payers must acknowledge health care as a longitudinal concern, not a temporary one. Long-term-contract models such have demonstrated improved clinical outcomes and cost savings. Longer contracts incentivize insurers to focus on preventive care and end-of-life decisions. Otherwise, when there is a commonly shared resource, every user or patient benefits from its use but shares the costs of its abuse.

Preventive Actions: When perceptions become embedded in assumptions and conflict, they lead to deep beliefs about the organization and its ability to be successful. At the system level, the behavior of health insurers could be characterized as the tragedy of the commons. For example, the cost of cure is front-loaded, but the benefits accrue over time. As such, insurers may attempt to delay treatment or avoid patients who require it, in the hope they might change insurers. Policy options to remedy this Commons problem must include alignment of incentives at the patient level, coordination among payers, and government intervention similar to pre-admission policies. Stakeholders need to collaborate to establish equitable mechanisms fairly distribute the cost and benefits of high-cost cures.[12] An approach would be to establish methods for making the cumulative effects of using the common resource more real and immediate. This approach would include evaluation of the Commons to determine options replace or substitute the resource before becoming obsolete.

Archetype -- Tragedy of the Commons (Continued)

Other preventive actions include educating others, so they understand the consequences of abusing the resource. This action also restores or strengthens the missing feedback link, either by privatizing the resource or letting the user experience the direct consequences of abuse. Another approach is to make the long-term effects more present, remove constraints, or establish policies on access to resources.

Health Leader Imperatives: Tragedy of the Commons is a classic example of reductionist thinking. Being unaware of the effect of the parts, on the whole, allows others to think and behave as though there are no organizational effects. Changes to the current health system must incorporate incentive structures. By not reconciling motivations with the best intentions, the U.S. health care system could continue to be unsustainable to the point of collapse.

Archetype -- Information Asymmetry –Special form of "Tragedy of the Commons."

Concept: Information Asymmetry is caused by trying to handle a problem at too low a level in the system, so it would seem sensible all problems be dealt with from the highest point of the system. For example, the medical care market flawed because of asymmetric information. The doctor knows more than the patient. As a result, providers recommend unnecessary care to enhance revenue streams even though no benefit accrues to patients. Providers may recommend one drug or device over another because of financial relations. Patients with limited knowledge have no reliable way of evaluating the quality of the advice they are getting. About the only check on the system is third-party payer utilization review. However, this is crude and highly imperfect activity engaged in by another party who has a financial interest in the outcome. In many respects, this level is reflective of the system level where comparative effectiveness, price and cost transparency is a policy issue. In another example, the employer-based insurance system makes this problem worse. When the employer pays premiums, individuals become more ignorant about just how much health care costs. Health care will cost an average 23-year-old at least $1.8 million over the course of his or her lifetime. However, individuals don't realize how high this number is because employers pay it. A large proportion of the $1.8 million could transfer back to taxpayers if health services were less expensive, but because the costs are hidden, individuals do not know they are losing out.[1] Also, individuals do not like to have everything controlled by Government, preferring to have some direct input into the decision-making process. The conflict here is twofold. Should control be given to the lowest level of the system which would be quicker, less costly and simpler, but full of its set of problems as illustrated above? Alternatively, should the control be given to the top end of the system, which might reduce conflicts between the subsystems, but cost more, be less efficient, and take longer to implement?

Preventive Actions: The best way to deal with this, according to Kauffman is to "make each decision at the lowest possible level, but be ready to shift the control of the situation to a higher level if a serious problem occurs."[9] For example, an option to fix the distortion of health insurance patients cold pay for it outright similar to other areas of life. A proposal could be to restrict insurance coverage to catastrophic costs—rare, unpredictable, serious illnesses—and pay for other care out of pocket. This proposal gives individuals the chance to pay for expensive treatments through insurance while giving them more information about the options and true costs of routine care. Putting consumers in the driver's seat revolutionizes health care and health insurance [1]. Natural systems do this automatically. Unless there is a problem with the heart or another internal organ, the body automatically knows to breathe, allow blood to flow, and move muscles. However, if something goes wrong in one of the systems in the body, the responsibility for repair goes to the rest of the body's system.[2] With man-made systems such as the economy or government, choosing a level at which to deal with problems is not at all automatic. Individuals can be ignorant about the problem until it is too late, or resentful of giving over power to the government. Moreover, even if they do give over control, they end up complaining and criticizing because they are unaware of the difficulty in getting rid of the imperfections in the system.[2]

Archetype -- Information Asymmetry – Special form of "Tragedy of the Commons." (Continued)

      A solution to this dilemma is to accept some sloppiness in a system. For instance, while selling illegal drugs is against the law, the government sometimes overlooks the minor dealers. The reason for this is it would cost too much to investigate every suspected dealer, and it would take away human resources and time from pursuing the larger scale drug transactions. It is more prudent, in this case, to allow for some sloppiness in the system so as to pursue more critical goals. This "sloppiness" does not mean governments should ignore problems like this. It does mean, however, no society can be perfect and solving one problem almost always creates another. The best option, therefore, is to accept some imperfection in the system.[2]

      <u>Health Leader Imperatives</u>: Individuals are increasingly faced with making healthcare choices based on limited information about the price and value of services. At the policy level, the Agency for Healthcare Research and Quality could be a central resource for consumers seeking health-care information and a group of well-trained professionals—medical decision advisers—could help individuals interpret highly technical health information.

Archetype -- Accidental Adversaries

Concept: Accidental Adversaries is similar to the Escalation archetype regarding the pattern of behavior develops over time. It is different insofar as the intent of the parties. Accidental Adversaries begin relations with win-win goals, generally taking advantage of their strengths with the objective of accomplishing the goals together. For example, when doctors are paid for performance, the more care they deliver, and the better they do financially. This perverseness leads to unnecessary tests and procedures making doctors the adversaries of their patients and health plan managers. Incentives are just as perverse with insurance plans. The less care they deliver, the more profit they make or the closer they stay to budget allocations. This situation makes accidental adversaries out of insurance or government and their clients or taxpayers.

The "offended" party perceives actions of others as gaining an unfair advantage in the partnership or harms the "offended" party (at worst). The spirit of partnership turns to one of the contentious adversaries. For example, the internal and external environments of health have become adversarial. Most systems have formed a defense against an increasingly hostile environment.[5] Patients expect answers for their problems and trained health professionals to have answers. These expectations often remain unfulfilled. The provider may not have the answer for a specific patient's problems because a correct answer with a guaranteed outcome for the patient does not exist [1]. Rather than engaging in dialogue, the offended party assumes they know everything about the action (including the foreknowledge it was willful and hostile), there is no point in discussing it, and their only option is to right the wrong. In fact, the first party may not know their actions are harmful to hurtful. When the second party responds, the first party makes the same assumptions. The first party's recourse? Retaliate. Once the adversarial relationship continues, the behavior is similar to the Escalation archetype. However, the outer reinforcing loop is still available should they suspend their mental models and engage in dialogue. The root of misunderstandings, unrealistic expectations, performance problems or mistakes can be revealed, giving the parties a fresh start.

Preventive Actions: Collaboration. Many cooperative efforts begin on a good note only to deteriorate over time, often as the need for collaboration deepens. This archetype should help parties collaborative to gain insight on how the actions are filtered to produce unintended interpretations. Other preventive measures were reviewing the original understanding and expected benefits and identifying conflicting incentives driving adversarial behavior. Finally, each party should develop overarching goals to align efforts, establish metrics to monitor collaborative behavior and establish regular communication.

> **Archetype -- Accidental Adversaries (Continued)**
>
> <u>Health Leader Imperatives</u>: The lesson of Accidental Adversaries lies in the power of mental models to supply all too quick explanations of situations. Unless judgment is suspended these mental models can drive one, both or all parties to conclusions bear a remote resemblance to the underlying reason the "breach" in the relationship occurred in the first place, if indeed any violation took place. The degree to which partners embrace a vision in common and articulate expectations is a significant contributor to tempering negativity. A shared vision will contribute to the extent partners engage in fixing problems in each other's organization. Shared Vision is connected to a sense of mission, purpose, values and culture. The vision must be the foundation of a partnership drawing attention to team learning. If the partners adopt a principle of continuous improvement and learning, the probability of success increases.

Reflection

Today's health system, a system with eroding goals and drifting to low performance must be refocused. The systems Archetypes are stories, and concepts representing pathologies or patterns of behavior emerge from underlying system structures. Until leaders quit rewarding A and hoping for B, nothing will change. Archetypes can be used to reveal insights into an existing structure or prospectively to anticipate potential problems and symptoms. Archetypes do not describe specific problems; they describe families of problems generically. Their value comes from insights into the dynamic interaction of complex systems especially outside one's stovepipes or expertise. As part of a suite of instruments, archetypes help develop understanding about an organization's environment and how they contribute to effectively solving problems at all levels. A provider who unilaterally spends more time with patients, a pharmaceutical company which unilaterally lowers prices, a hospital whom reduces re-admit rate, or a hospital CEO who skipped the purchase of a shiny new edifice to invest high-reliability care processes would be punished economically and professionally for doing what was right. Archetypes facilitate change at all levels.

Also, systems archetypes can be a major component of strategic planning. Strategies can be tested using archetypes to identify potential pitfalls and address them in the planning stages when they are easier to tackle. Systems archetypes provide mental models and language to communicate how an organization is not and should be performing without blame. Having the mental imagery and language to document, communicate, and analyze behaviors provides a useful framework for dealing with change, preventing, or eliminate negative behavioral patterns. Once the nuances of systems archetypes are mastered, this knowledge can be leveraged to build robust systems capable of generating sustainable solutions while reducing pathologies.

Part III: APPLICATIONS

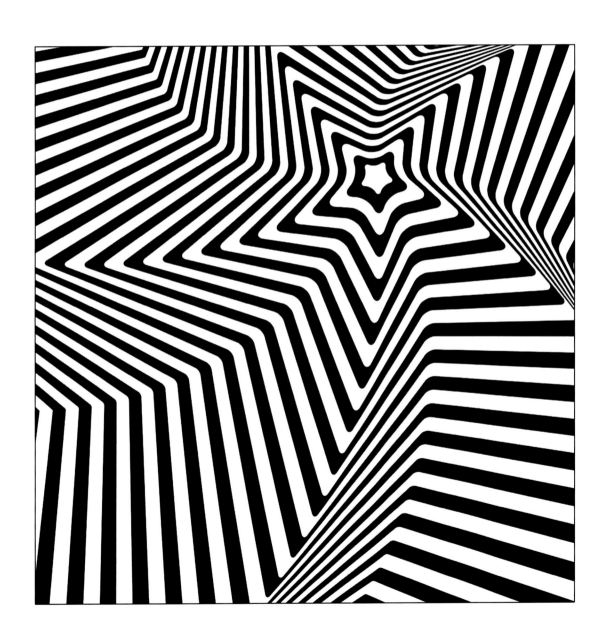

Overview of Part III

Part III challenges leaders to see the forest [systems] for the trees [parts] and the fragility of the ecosystem [sum of all connections]" in the form of "composite" case studies. The case studies illustrate the need to work with many actors and stakeholders to generate sustainable solutions rather than attractive fixes that may later fail or decline into dysfunction. When superficial symptoms of complex problems are addressed, underlying problems remain unsolved, these problems are exacerbated with the "solutions" feeding a vicious cycle. An example is managed care which was touted as the answer for US healthcare with reduced cost and improved quality of care strategies only to exacerbate recurring problems by creating newer problems later.

Part III illustrates the applications of methods, tools and mental models by utilizing the application of methods and tools from **Part II**. The variety of case studies is provided in different settings and in the context of the levels of systems. These systems thinking applications should challenge leaders, policy analysts, planners, and strategists to focus on processes, interactions and causes of poor outcomes, focusing on sustainable solutions rather than interim results. Application of systems thinking must be considered in the context of other competencies such as active listening, aspirational and critical thinking, and collaboration or networking across organizational boundaries. However, those competencies should not overshadow the use of a systems approach to understanding complex systems dynamics and generating sustainable solutions. Many health organizations attempt to be their own islands, as closed, self-contained systems. An impossible goal, since health systems at any level are living systems. For example, a primary care system is a subsystem within a community health system impacting the social determinants of health. This way of thinking challenges the reader to begin reframing the problem, understanding the frames of reference and perspectives of the various actors and stakeholders to approach any problem differently with the application of systems thinking methods and tools. Furthermore, the reader will see how the benefits of using an actor and stakeholder approach as part of systems thinking are numerous. First, the opinions of stakeholders shape solutions and improve the likelihood of sustainability. By communicating with stakeholders early and frequently, health systems leaders can ensure they fully understand what is at stake and the benefits of an initiative. Second, gaining support facilitates access to resources. Finally, as systems thinkers, anticipating a stakeholder's reaction and interests will support acquiring their support.

Chapter 10: Understanding Frames of Reference in the Context of a Opioid Crisis

The US opioid crisis is a serious public health issue affecting millions of individuals across the country. Drug overdose deaths are the leading cause of injury-related death in the United States. The crisis shows no signs of stopping. Local actors and stakeholders are paralyzed over the sheer complexity of the problem. In 2014, more individuals died from drug overdoses than in previous years. The majority of these deaths (more than six out of ten) involved an opioid.

The pace of addiction and death is so fast in some locations the statistics are overwhelming. Since 1999, the overdose rates involving opioids including prescription pain relievers and heroin almost quadrupled. Over 165,000 individuals died from prescription opioid overdoses since 1999. An increase in heroin-involved deaths and deaths involving synthetic opioids was recorded in 2014.[127] According to Institute of Healthcare Improvement's (IHI) research highlights the following gaps:

- Absence of health systems in many community coalitions
- Absence of law enforcement, corrections, and social services in others and coordination with health and public health organizations
- Shortage of detoxification beds and addiction treatment facilities
- Poor cross over and continuity between detoxification and addiction treatment, which is the most critical time to prevent a fatal overdose.[128]

Effective community wide interventions are needed. However, the complexity of the opioid crisis requires multiple actors and stakeholders: medical, legislative, behavioral, educational, and legal changes working together to understand the depth of the problem so a sustainable solution can be coordinated with communities, state, and federal levels.[129] Addressing this epidemic requires a systems thinking approach to engage different stakeholders and methods to reverse the trends. While systems thinking is necessary, understanding frames of reference or perspectives of actors and stakeholders is also imperative.[128]

Understanding Frames of Reference as a Systems Thinking Skill

When health system and community leaders transform from an isolationist frame of reference to a systems thinking mindset, integrating multiple perspectives becomes obvious to understanding systemic problems and solutions. This transition is especially critical when determining the best methods and tools for a given situation. For example, integration or augmentation of systems thinking approaches and continuous quality improvement and strategic planning in the context of creating high-reliability health organizations is becoming more common, but not universal enough to reduce the number of preventable deaths. The opioid crisis is treated no different from other health policy approaches other than the set of non-health and health leaders is larger. However, a systems thinking mindset must transition to the community as well.

The power of systems thinking is derived from integrating multiple perspectives to the situation being analyzed. For example, global health systems strengthening initiatives are beginning to emerge as blueprints in the application of systems thinking methods and tools to create sustainable solutions at the local, region, and country levels with minimal unintended consequences. Solving the opioid crisis will require challenging deeply held assumptions, overcoming blame, developing and experimenting with a variety of solutions, and sharing the lessons learned everywhere and anywhere.

Just as important, there is validity and value in viewing problems from another perspective especially those of community stakeholders. For example, the local and county opioid crises contain multiple solutions and policy implications, however, understanding the multiple perspectives, often contradicting and contrived from the different levels is critical. Capturing the perspectives of actors and stakeholders is a necessary skill in applying systems thinking concepts, methods, and tools. Differing perspectives or angles may arise from the different interests, backgrounds, and experiences of the stakeholders. For example framing or reframing the opioid crises from a demand or supply driven problem drives different solutions? Viewing the problem as a treatment or prevention issue is based on value and resources. Determining how the crisis can be solved quickly and sooner rather than later will be a major challenge.

Multiple Perspectives

Solving the opioid crisis will take a community-wide effort and work at the national, state, and local levels to adequately address the problem. Shifting the burden to a few agencies may be an option, however it is not likely to be efficacious. The simplest approach is to consider the interests or positions of the actors and stakeholders during the problem assessment. Health systems leaders should be neutral and work to see and understand stakeholder perspectives and attitudes. Researchers have identified critical components to developing a system-wide community solution.[128] It begins with an acknowledgement of a systems approach and everyone in the community has a role.

Multiple perspectives can be assessed and mapped when the stakeholder community is available for interviews and focus groups. When interactions with the actors and stakeholders are limited, consulting with subject matter experts is an alternative, albeit less desirable. The systems thinkers must place themselves in the role of each actor and stakeholder and assesses the problem considering the stakeholders' concerns and needs. An alternative technique is to approach problem analysis from the perspective of different disciplines. A facilitator may choose to view the problem from the lens of a scientist, technologist, business person, and social worker.[130,131] However, the risk here is that the development of solutions may be one-sided or marginal. For example, restriction of prescription drugs with regulatory mechanisms may increase deaths, just as the war on illegal drugs has. As such, this approach forces the systems practitioner to expand their point of view and address the problem situation from a system-wide angle. Those who produce or prescribe opioids, treat addiction, enforce the law, educate others, family members, and individuals taking opioids have a role. The table below shows high-level and specific actions, along with the principal actors and stakeholders required to implement a coordinated, systematic approach across a community.[129]

Table 3
Applications, Actions, Actors and Stakeholder Opioids Crisis

High-level Applications	Specific Actions	Actors and Stakeholders

Reduce stigma	• Provide education for:
	  o Providers and health teams
	  o Individuals, families, and relatives
	  o Law enforcement agencies at all levels
		• Auxiliary provider and services
		• Public school system
		• Public Health Organizations
		• Law enforcement (treatment not just crime)

Prevent death from overdose	• Administer Naloxone and another drug • Increase availability of Naloxone in community • Educate family, friends, associates on signs of overdose and use of specific drugs	• Emergency Medical Technicians (EMT), clinicians, law enforcement • Legislative • Legislative, Individual, Provider
Manage opioid-dependent population	• Taper patients from high-dose, chronic use • Educate patients, families, friends about pain management • Increase availability and monetary reimbursement of alternative pain management therapies	• Providers • Providers • Payers or Insurers
Link detoxification and ongoing treatment and recovery services	• Provide current MAT when appropriate • Provide ongoing group therapy • Implement drug courts	• Providers • Providers, payers or Insurers, Peer support • Attorney General, law enforcement
Increase availability of non-opioid alternatives for chronic pain management such as acupuncture	• Change reimbursements policies • Educate providers and health teams on effective, alternative pain management strategies and follow-up tactics	• Payers: private and public • Requires academic and teaching guidelines, requirements, and education/implementation
Identify opioid-addicted individuals and patients	• Assess for substance abuse disorder at clinic and health team, or physician visits • Use guidelines and alerts to identify opioid-seeking patients	• Law enforcement, EMTs, Providers, Pharmacists • Providers and Health Teams, Allied Health Professionals, and Public and Community Health teams

High-level Applications	Specific Actions	Actors and Stakeholders
Enroll in extensive substance abuse treatment services	• Improve and increase availability of inpatient detoxification services • Improve and increase availability of outpatient detoxification services • Train health teams to use Medication-Assisted Treatment (MAT) procedures, and processes • Increase availability of MAT trained professionals • Increase availability of Behavioral Health services such as integration with primary care services	• Providers, law enforcement, EMTs, public health, payers
Educate about risks of prescription opioids	• Identify patients at greater risk for addiction • Inform the public about the danger of prescription opioids and other destructive drugs	• Providers Education, Public Health
Reduce availability of recreational opioids	• Prosecute dealer to the maximum extent by classifying overdose death as crimes versus unusual deaths • Change classification of controlled substances • Arrest and prosecute dealers	• Attorney General Attorney General, legislation • Detention or law enforcement agencies at all levels
Reduce supplies of prescription and street level opioids	• Change prescribing practices (e.g. dose, duration, reason, limit, requirement for follow-up) with clinical practice guidelines • Change dispensing practices to include double verification • Prevent diversion of the goal of better health and recovery • Limit pharmaceutical production and misleading advertisements	• Set up coalition of health teams, medical group practices, and national or state legislative collaborative • Pharmacists, Payers, legislation • Patients, health and non-health community organizations (safe drug disposal or drop off points) • National legislative measures, FDA, pharmaceutical companies

High-level Applications	Specific Actions	Actors and Stakeholders
Decrease demand for recreational opioid use	• Implement drug courts • Eliminate pre-authorization for SA treatment • Build robust recovery system	• Attorney General • Attorney General, payers • Public health, behavioral health services
Create faster learning and reinforcing feedback loops or knowledge sharing networks	• Report opioid overdoses to any provider linked to the individual without fear of blame or reprisal • Provide access for all to Prescription Drug Monitoring Program (PDMP) and other guidelines • Use PDMP and other guidelines at each patient encounter	• Medical examiner • State legislation • Medical societies, provider networks, Public Health

Adapted by D. Anderson from Martin L, Laderman A Systems Approach Is The Only Way To Address The Opioid Crisis, Health Affairs Blog. 7500 Old Georgetown Road, Suite 600, Bethesda, MD 20814-6133: Health Affairs Blog; 2016

Seeing and Anticipating Short Versus Long Term Solutions

Seeing both short and long term means seeing with both eyes (open). Health leaders applying systems thinking position themselves so they can see and anticipate the forest *and* the trees with respect to this crisis. Systems thinkers must be generic and specific simultaneously. They must also envision the human dynamic in the patterns of behavior and associated events.[132] When the systems thinker is comfortable with an understanding of one aspect of a problem, understanding opposing views and challenging their personal assumptions adds depth and completeness to the assessment.

The health systems thinking leader must assess and understand the extremes, the opposites, and the opposing perspectives. This approach requires the skill to simplify the complex through inquiry, synthesis, and analysis as well as active listening. For example, community and state level actors and stakeholders will succeed if they align local actors to create community systems to prevent new individuals from becoming dependent on opioids while supporting recovery simultaneously. Failing to take such this approach results apathy and more stress among those striving to improve the situation.[129]

Seeing Beyond the Linear Relations and Organization Walls

Seeing interrelationships between processes and the parts of the linear cause-effect chains is an integral systems thinking skill. Untouched linear processes or chains of events result from a high degree of comfortableness with the status quo. They are the product of a lack of deep understanding, exposure or perhaps dysfunctional thinking caused by isolation from the challenge. The health systems thinker understands when differing perspectives are not independent events, but are related and reinforce the problem—reinforcing and balancing loops.

In the case of opioid addition, actions are being taken at several levels to prevent addiction and treat those who are. The Center for Disease Control and Prevention's (CDC) guidelines, for example, help provider and health teams prescribe opioids appropriately, responsibly, and ethically. The Department of Health and Human Services (DHHS)' recently recommend increasing patient treatment load limits from 100 to 200 patients as a measure to help health provider teams. The limit allows more individuals to receive the treatment they need to end their dependence on opioids within the CDC's guidelines.[129] State level actors and stakeholders are implementing other structural solutions such as drug courts, teams of narcotics detectives and emergency medical technicians (EMTs) to be trusted case managers helping guide individuals to voluntary treatment rather than incarceration. Many medical examiners serve as health team educators when overdoses occur. Again, although these efforts are underway, they are not sufficient to reverse this crisis.[129]

Detail Complexity vs. Dynamic Complexity as Frames of Reference

When assessing today's opioid crisis, it is easy to be overwhelmed by complexity. Systems thinkers feel compelled to provide more complex solutions. This temptation should be resisted. Instead, systems thinkers should seek to reduce the problem to the simplest acceptable form. To do so requires differentiating between detail complexity and dynamic complexity, both being equally important.[133]

Detail complexity is the airplane with many parts or the machine assembly with many steps. Leaders do not need to know intimate details about the system or its behavior. They do, however, need to conduct an end-to-end assessment of the major system parts and their relations. Dynamic complexity is related to system behavior and how the system interacts with the external environment and within the parts. This approach includes assessing how the parts work together-- their formal or informal relationships, why they work or don't work together, and how they react to surprises. Understanding the bigger movements throughout the system is essential to system assessment.

Detail versus dynamic complexity may be easier to manage once the system of actors and stakeholder roles and responsibilities are captured and fully transparent. Managing interventions related to coordination, logistics, promotion, and resources has considerable detail complexity in solving the opioid crisis. However, seeing how the parts work together makes uncovering leverage points, identifying quick wins, and overall implementation easier. Since the impact and evolution of the opioid crisis, there is considerable dynamic complexity as well. The system must be robust and agile enough to account for unanticipated needs, programs whose capacity has been exceeded, and behavioral change. In many cases, communities are often resource-rich, and coordination is poor. Resources such as financial, human, information systems, and infrastructure are precious. Given the extent of the opioid crisis, they cannot be wasted. Unlikely partners must learn to work together, communicate continuously, and think beyond their usual boundaries or personal interests.

Well-intentioned health service providers need to work together across organizations, thus, moving beyond the borders of their institutions and traditional roles and rules to create new relationships and pathways to provide coordinated services to those in need.[129] Approximately 75 percent of heroin users started on the road to addiction with prescription drugs. Leaders, actors, and stakeholders can reframe the conversation with patients and families with a discussion on how prescription opioids affect the human anatomy especially the brain.[129] Actors and stakeholders should communicate that many of those who became addicted to prescription opioids did not approach the use of opioids as a purely recreational activity. They were taking medication to relieve pain as prescribed by their physician or perhaps to self-medicate emotional issues. Proper use of opioids should be much more limited than it currently is.[129] This approach may require retraining of health teams and providers to reduce the risk of receiving misinformation about the risks of prescription opioids. Changing a practice takes time. Effective alternatives for chronic pain management requires both providers and payers to provide the right incentives to apply them.[129]

External Frame of Reference

A distance view frame of reference provides the big picture, i.e. the ability to see the forest for the trees. All systems problems must be viewed from afar without bias to seeing the interdependent components and intricate relationships such as handoffs between entities.[132] By focusing too narrowly, the assessment may miss pivotal aspects of the system behavior. For example, while many promising ideas are evidence-informed, many have not been rigorously evaluated. The urgent need for action requires rapid implementation, careful evaluation of other promising policies and programs. This requires a holistic approach and innovative solutions--that need to be supported.[134] Comprehensive interventions must include the whole system involving interventions supported by the supply chain, local clinics, and community addiction treatment settings. Sustainable solutions must be implemented to prevent individuals from progressing down a pathway to misuse, abuse, addiction, and overdose. Therefore primary, secondary and tertiary prevention strategies are vital. The importance of creating synergies and alignment across different organizations and respective interventions to maximize available resources is critical.[134]

Internal Frame of Reference

If a problem is resistant to change then the common solution or the underlying system itself could be the problem. This issue is one of the core premises in systems thinking. The internal frame of reference leads someone to think the internal working parts of the system are the cause of dysfunctionality. The systems thinker may view the system structure as the root cause of the problem rather than seeing the patterns as influenced by internal and external agents.[132] Community level solutions with motivated actors and stakeholders are imperative. For example, used appropriately, prescription opioids can provide relief to patients. However, these therapies are often prescribed in quantities or for conditions considered excessive beyond evidence-based guidelines. These practices lack the attention needed for safe prescribing, storage, and disposal of drugs. Lack of awareness and misinformation has also contributed to misuse, abuse, addiction, and overdose cases occurring the past ten years. Efforts to maximize a favorable risk and benefit balance of prescription opioids are best achieved through a prudent, yet judicial application of clinical practice guidelines.[134] A more balanced approach should focus on local solutions to develop prescribing guidelines, implement drug monitoring programs, train pharmacy benefit leaders and pharmacists on indicators of abuse, establish addiction treatment centers, and implement community-based prevention and awareness programs.[134]

Multiple Frames of Reference

Multiple perspectives or frames of reference are an essential part of the systems thinking process especially when the complexity of a challenge such as the opioid crisis. Prescription drugs including opioids are essential to improving the quality of life for many living with acute or chronic pain. However, misuse, abuse, addiction, and overdose trends must be reversed as a serious public health problem. A systemic and comprehensive response to this crisis must focus on prevention and improve processes associated with new addiction. This approach requires earlier identification and referral of opioid-addicted individuals and ensuring access to effective opioid addiction treatment services.[134] Actors and stakeholders, including clinicians, researchers, government officials, injury prevention professionals, law enforcement leaders, pharmaceutical manufacturers and distributors, lawyers, health insurers and patient representatives must be part of the solution.[134] Health systems thinking can serve as the "method out of the madness" in this challenging and increasingly global crisis.

To have a solid understanding of a problem situation, the systems thinker must understand as many actor and stakeholder perspectives as possible. Addicted individuals or families of those who are addicted or who have died, come from all segments of society and all parts of the globe. Addiction is a psychological and physical condition and recovery is long and difficult. Unfortunately, stigma often prevents individuals from seeking help sooner rather than later.[129] It is imperative the health systems leaders and policymakers look at the problem situation in multiple ways and through multiple lenses. Many addiction and crisis reduction efforts focus on silver bullet solutions. Community health and leaders cannot focus prescribing guidelines, distribution, or increased access to treatment and prevention services in isolation. Leaders must connect actors and stakeholders to a master plan because of the interconnected nature of the problem. Preventing fatal overdoses is important, but addressing the ongoing addiction crisis necessarily requires a systems approach.[129]

Chapter 11: Ending Homelessness --- Stock-n-Flow and Causal Loop Diagrams

For city officials, community leaders, and health providers, placing homeless individuals in shelters is the most inexpensive and human way to meet the basic needs of individuals experiencing homelessness. Some may even believe shelters are an ideal solution. However, are they? Healthy People 2020 as highlighted in figure below highlights the importance of the social determinants of health or circumstances where individuals are born, live, work, and age. It also highlights the systems they use to deal with a crisis, security, and illnesses. Health starts in the individual's homes, schools, workplaces, neighborhoods, and communities.

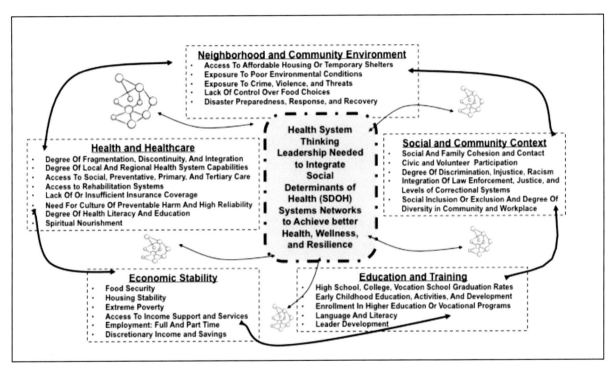

Part 3, Chapter 11, Figure 19: Social Determinants Of Health in Relation To Homelessness. Adapted by D. Anderson

Homelessness or unstable housing represents a significant social determinant of health. Accommodations and employment are two social determinants of health that work hand-in-hand, both significantly impacting health outcomes. The conditions in which individuals live explain why some Americans are healthier than others or not as healthy as they could be. The social determinants of health within Healthy People 2020 are designed to identify ways to create social and physical environments promote good health for all.[135] Unemployed individuals are likely to self-report worse health status, may experience more depressive symptoms, and are at a higher risk for mortality.[136] Unfortunately, homelessness contributes to poor health and prosperity for individuals and communities.

Most likely, homeless patients may be predisposed to worse health outcomes compared to other patients due to poor living conditions, psychosocial stress, and food insecurity. Additionally, these patients tend to have limited resources for self-care and utilize health services more than their counterparts. According to the Agency for Healthcare Research and Quality (AHRQ), rates of emergency department visits were nine times higher among homeless single men, 12 times higher among homeless single women, and 3.4 times higher among homeless adults in families compared to the study's control parameters. Hospitalization rates were 8.5 times higher among homeless single males, 4.6 times higher among homeless single women, and 2.1 times higher among homeless adults in families. Health care utilization "outliers" were far more prevalent and more extreme among homeless participants, particularly for non-ambulatory care compared to the control population. The maximum annual number of emergency department encounters was 108 per year for the homeless group, compared to 14 per year in the control group.[137]

Compared to the housed population, individuals without homes experience increased mortality, chronic health conditions, mental illness, substance use, and engage in risky health behaviors. The homeless are more likely to face poverty resulting in an inability to maintain a residence, pay for healthcare, and afford daily necessities like food and clothing.[135] For example, a homeless patient with diabetes may have difficulty managing their condition due to a lack of a storage place for their insulin or due to poor access to nutritious food [136]. The health costs of the homeless can be high. Hospitalization, treatment, incarceration, police intervention and emergency shelter expenses add up making homelessness expensive for communities and taxpayers. According to a *New England Journal of Medicine* report, the homeless spent an average of four days longer per hospital visit than a comparable non-homeless patient. This extra cost, about $2,414 per hospitalization, is attributable to homelessness.[138] Similarly, a study of hospital admissions of homeless individuals in Hawaii indicated 1,751 adults were responsible for 564 hospitalizations or $4 million in costs. Their rate of psychiatric hospitalization was 100 times higher than their non-homeless cohort. The researchers conducting the study estimated the excess cost for treating homeless individuals was $3.5 million or about $2,000 per person.[139]

Homelessness crosses many civilian and governmental sectors at all levels. For example, a study examined health service utilization and costs for homeless and domiciled veterans hospitalized in psychiatric and substance abuse units at all Department of Veterans Affairs (VA) medical centers. Of the 9,108 veterans surveyed, 20% had been homeless at the time of admission; 15% of the veterans had doubled in shelters for a total homelessness rate of 35%. After adjusting for other factors, the average annual cost of care for homeless veterans was $27,206. Twenty-six percent of annual inpatient VA mental health expenditures are spent on the care of the homeless veteran. Homelessness adds to the cost of health care services for veterans with mental illness in VA. These results are most likely similar for other "safety net" systems serving the poor.[140] The challenge of ending homelessness is complex, to say the least. Systems thinking can apply to develop a shared understanding of why chronic, complex problems exist – as well as where leverage points are to solve problems in sustainable ways.

Homelessness both causes and can result from acute health care issues, including addiction, psychological disorders, HIV/AIDS, and a host of order ailments that can require long-term, consistent care. This inability to treat medical problems can aggravate these problems, making them both more dangerous and more costly.[141] As an example, physician and health care experts determined the average cost to cure an alcohol-related illness is approximate $10,660.[142]

Another study found the average cost to California hospitals of treating a substance abuse is about $8,360 for those in treatment, and $14,740 for those who are not.[142] Homelessness inhibits care, and housing instability detracts from regular medical attention, access to treatment, and recuperation.

Using Stock and Flow and Causal Loop Diagrams

Approximately 3 million Americans experience homelessness annually. Parents with children account for one-fifth of the homeless population. The homeless suffer from high rates of illness, frequently encounter barriers to accessing care, and use the health system at higher rates.[137] This composite case study illustrates how a community's "Homeless Coalition" addressed chronic homelessness surrounding a County-X. By applying systems thinking tools such as stock and flow and causality diagrams and discussing perspectives and the frames of reference of multi-sector stakeholders the community designed a ten-year initiative leading change with a lasting social impact.

Despite County-X's efforts, City-X with a population of 100,000 individuals could not solve the homelessness problem. Service providers, business and political leaders, policy analysts, and even homeless individuals themselves asked, "Why, have we been unable to end homelessness?" The problem with ending homelessness is not about lack of knowledge or availability of best practices, rather more about community actors and stakeholders developing a shared vision based on system dynamics underlying homelessness and establishing common goals with leverage points for transforming the current community based system.[143]

By using interview and focus groups and application of systems thinking tools, the participants captured the size and interconnectedness of the problem. The team clarified the disincentives for change, and helped each team see their responsibility to achieve the desired state from their perspectives.

Through the use of stock and flow and causality loop diagrams, the analysis identified a scenario in four steps:

1. Four stages of homelessness are summarized in the stock and flow diagram below. They are becoming at risk losing a home, losing home and having to live on the streets, finding temporary shelter off the streets, moving from a temporary shelter back into permanent housing.

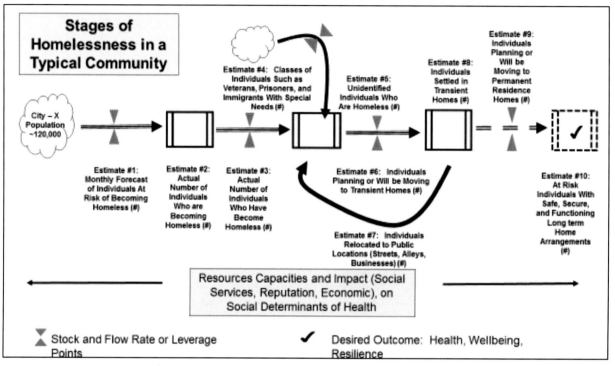

Part 3, Chapter 11, Figure 20: Illustration Of Stages Of Homelessness With Stock And Flow Rates Or Leverage Points For Policy Intervention. Adapted by D. Anderson from Stroh DP, Goodman, Michael. A Systemic Approach to Ending Homelessness. Applied Systems Thinking Journal. 2007;4

2. <u>Risks Result in Homelessness</u> are individual risk factors (i.e., health, safety, shelter), limited permanent, accessible, living wage jobs, financial problems (medical emergencies, child support, rent), limited permanent, safe, affordable, supportive housing, and social risks (aging, meth lab startups). The impact of these risk factors increased over time as the ability to find ethical landlords and affordable housing decreased. Faced with added financial challenges of renting to individuals at risk for homelessness, well-intentioned landlords, worried about their livelihood reduced the availability of affordable housing thus creating more homelessness. Community organizations attempted to prevent individuals from losing their homes. State and social services agencies provided emergency responses. The government provided subsidies. Family, friends, churches, and schools offered support. Many provided information about available resources. Also, the Veterans Affairs (VA) offered transitional support to veterans. Unfortunately, the assistance was not enough to create momentum with these solutions. Many individuals fell into the homelessness cycle or resorted to many living arrangements among friends and relatives, hidden from social services providers and the public.[143] County- X is also home to a Veterans

Health Administration (VHA) psychiatric hospital. Veterans throughout the state came to City-X for short and long-term treatment. Many of the veterans decided to stay in the area without housing, living on the streets, or in shelters.

3. <u>Why People get Off the Streets Only Temporarily</u>: Short-term options to get off the streets included 30-day shelters. Some homeless individuals ended up back on the street, emergency rooms, jail, or in unsafe housing. Many recycled through the temporary solutions for years. Case management was a limited resource, so the homeless received limited support. Many of the homeless cited self-determination as an important factor in overcoming adversity; however, a strong self-determination was insufficient without an infrastructure and services or a structure to secure permanent, safe, and affordable housing and living wage jobs.[143]

4. <u>What Prevented Individuals from Permanent Housing Arrangements</u>: Many leaders' recognized needed elements of sustainable solutions such as availability, awareness, and accessibility too much needed human services (i.e., detox, substance abuse treatment, and mental health services; discharge and transition planning for prisoners, life skills training, transitional housing; education, job training, and employment support). These solutions included the availability of permanent, safe, affordable, and supportive housing, living wage jobs and access to childcare and transportation services. Most important, the community's organic solutions were limited by several factors, including:

    - Time delays in implementing a solution and waiting for results (i.e., expectation of quick fixes versus long-term sustainable solutions)
    - Barriers produced by homelessness (e.g. legal identity, poor credit history, evictions, criminal record, negative stereotyping).
    - Ability to create permanent, living wage jobs and support

A complete picture of the system dynamics is presented in the figure below. These perceptions, barriers, and obstacles (vicious balancing loops) led to difficulties in individuals being unable to take advantage of available resources preventing them from moving to permanent housing. For example, communities limited individual's opportunity to improve their life skills and created reluctance on the part of landlords and employers to provide a new start. An unintended consequence of temporary shelters and support reduced the visibility of the problem to the community. Many individuals were fearful of being seen and thus hid their conditions. The lack of visibility reduced pressure in the community to solve the problem. The overnight success of shelters create pressure from donors to see short-term success and suppressed funding to innovate and collaborate including the use of existing resources for other initiatives.[143]

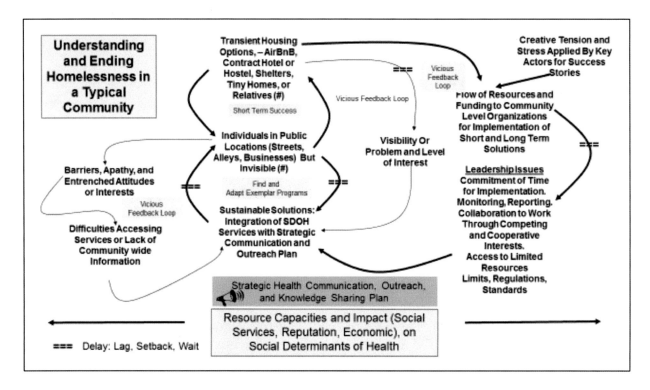

Part 3, Chapter 11, Figure 21: Balancing And Reinforcing Loops To Illustrate Homelessness In A Typical Community. Adapted by D. Anderson from Stroh DP, Goodman, Michael. A Systemic Approach to Ending Homelessness. Applied Systems Thinking Journal. 2007;4

Unfortunately, the overnight success led to:

- Fragmentation and lack of awareness of services
- Competition for existing funds and resources (or lack of utilization)
- Lack of broader knowledge of best practices
- Reluctance to overcome government restrictions
- Shelter as "the solution" mentality

These dynamics or balancing loops represent a familiar dynamic of shifting the burden (to the quick fix) or in psychological terms as "addiction" found in many complex social systems where a quick fix undermines sustainable solutions.[17]

Leverage Points

Several leverage points or types of interventions could help end homelessness. In this case study, two major interventions were identified. The figure below provides a visual of increasing and accelerating the number of individuals moving from temporary shelters into permanent housing and decreasing the number of individuals at risk from becoming homeless in the first place.[143]

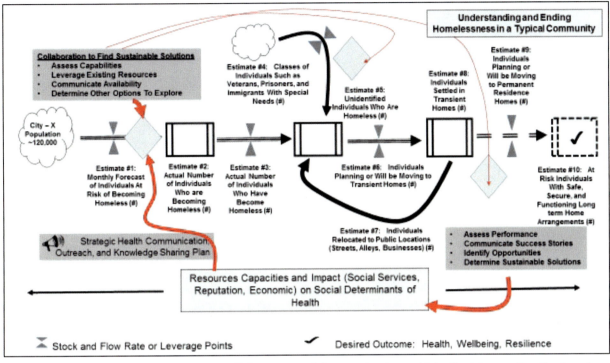

Part 3, Chapter 11, Figure 22: Applying Collaboration and Communication to Make Decisions at Key Stock and Flow Points. Adapted by D. Anderson from Stroh DP, Goodman, Michael. A Systemic Approach to Ending Homelessness. Applied Systems Thinking Journal. 2007;4

Moving People from Temporary to Permanent Housing: First, the coalition chose to increase the visibility of the problem as the first leverage point. This first step involved providing accurate information about the extent of the problem and the community's motivation to permanently solve it. Second, collaboration, alignment and investment among providers and community centered on reducing fragmentation and lack of awareness of services, limiting a shelter mentality, increasing knowledge of best practices, and willingness to overcome government restrictions to innovate was viewed as critical. For example, the local health system established stable primary care services modeled after the patient-centered medical home (PCMH) suited for homeless patients as part of a Federally Qualified Healthcare Center (FQHC). The services included walk-in visits only, team care to include behavioral health providers and social services team members, mobile and on-foot units, and access to a local shelter and medical respite program for post-hospital transitions within walking distance.[136] Finally, increasing access to permanent, safe, affordable, and supportive housing followed by access to substance abuse and mental health treatment for specific populations, and focus on partnerships to focus on economic development would lead to increased availability and access to living wage jobs.[143]

Designing a System to Prevent Homelessness: The least expensive interventions prevented individuals from being homeless in the first place. The leverage points included increasing affordable housing, jobs, and critical services to enable individuals at risk to keep their homes. Some approaches to help individuals retain their existing homes included supporting landlords to rent to individuals at risk so landlords would be able to maintain or even increase the stock of affordable homes. Solutions related to employment included the creation of sufficient living wage jobs to individual's ability to pay their rent.[143]

As homelessness and unemployment persist in the country and around the world, community health leaders should look to these examples of systems thinking to provide comprehensive care, improve health outcomes, and reduce health costs. In the case of homelessness, a health, social, and economic issue, making these advances involves working together, establishing shared goals, and maximizing opportunities for collaboration at all levels. Systems thinking, when integrated with community approaches to foster collaboration enables actors and stakeholders to move from misperceptions to an understanding of best practices to a shared commitment to creating community-wide sustainable solutions.[143]

Chapter 12: Using Causal Loops to Reduce Neonatal Mortality in Uganda

This study facilitates the understanding of the causes of neonatal mortality and the application of systems thinking methods and tools. The study explores the dynamics arising from neonatal health delivery complexity, non-linear thinking, and the interplay of public and social health systems factors, using Uganda as a case study.[144] Three million babies die annually within their first four weeks of life (neonatal period). Virtually all (99%) of the deaths occur in low-and-middle-income countries (LMICs). Global trends in neonatal mortality have shown alarmingly slow progress, the slowest being in sub-Saharan Africa. Three-quarters of the neonatal deaths occurred within the first week of life; at least 1 million die on day one of their life. Uganda is a high-burden country in sub-Saharan Africa. Child survival programs tend to focus on pneumonia, diarrhea, malaria, and vaccine-preventable diseases. While all of these situations contributed to death after the first month of life, targeted approaches to prevent death before birth and the first week of life have gone unrecorded.[145] Of the newborns who die annually, Uganda ranks the fifth highest in neonatal mortality rates or 43,000 neonatal deaths each year. Despite child survival and safe motherhood programs towards reducing infant mortality, insufficient attention has been given to this critical first month of life. There is an urgent need to employ alternative solutions to account for the intricate complexities of neonatal health and the health system.[144] The study utilized a dynamic synthesis methodology (DSM) to provide alternative solutions to problems. The figure below summarizes the current system.

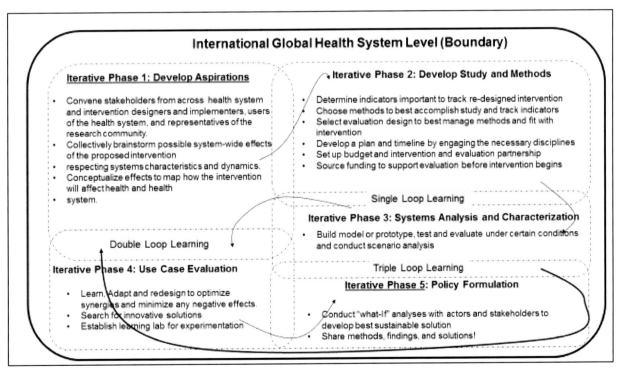

Part 3, Chapter 12, Figure 23: Initial Planning For Systems Thinking Case in Uganda. Adapted by D. Anderson from Rwashana AS, Nakubulwa, Sarah, Nakakeeto-Kijjambu, Margaret, Adam, Taghreed Advancing The Application Of Systems Thinking In Health: Understanding The Dynamics Of Neonatal Mortality In Uganda. Health Research Policy and Systems. 2014;12(36):1478-4505

The study began with a visual and was refined and validated using Causal Loop Diagrams (CLD). Application of systems thinking principles was conducted with interviews in the Kampala district with high neonatal mortality rates with mothers, social support systems, family, facilities, policymakers, and frontline health workers. To explain the system dynamics--interactions, interrelationships, and effects—generated by the data analysis and brainstorming sessions, a series of causal loop diagrams (CLDs) ranging from basic to complex depicted the causes of neonatal mortality. Later, the results were validated by local and international stakeholders.[144] CLDs facilitated understanding and depiction of the feedback mechanisms generated within complex systems: relationships, dynamics, and delays associated with the variables make them. Influence is shown by an arrow and an indicator on whether affected element changed in the same (+) or opposite (-) direction as the influencing element. A link from element A to element B ($A \xrightarrow{+} B$) may be positive if a change in A produces changes in the same direction, or negative ($A \xrightarrow{-} B$) if changes in A produces changes in B in the opposite direction. A change in element A producing a change in element B only after a delay is denoted $A \xrightarrow{||} B$.

The figure below shows a balancing loop whose goal is to increase the mothers' participation in health services and educational offerings. When more mothers participate the workload increases leading to increased wait times. The increased wait times result in frustration resulting in less participation. These reinforcing loops represent growing actions adding to another loop.

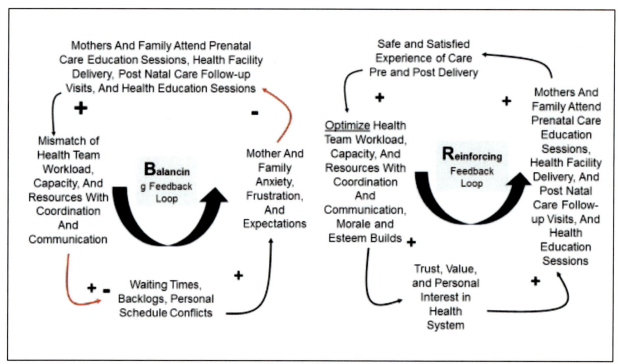

Part 3, Chapter 12, Figure 24: Illustration of Balancing and Reinforcing Loops. Adapted by D. Anderson from Rwashana AS, Nakubulwa, Sarah, Nakakeeto-Kijjambu, Margaret, Adam, Taghreed Advancing The Application Of Systems Thinking In Health: Understanding The Dynamics Of Neonatal Mortality In Uganda. Health Research Policy and Systems. 2014;12(36):1478-4505

These loops may be referred to as virtuous cycles when they produce desirable effects or vicious cycles when they produce adverse cycles. The figure also shows a reinforcing loop where participation in health services arising from safe deliveries results in more trust thus increasing more participation.

The team developed two Causal Loop Diagrams (CLDs) for supply and demand health issues. The CLDs are depicting the factors associated with neonatal mortality such as maternal health, the level of awareness of maternal and newborn health concerns, and availability of quality of services, among others.[144] Further, validation of the CLDs and underlying conceptual thinking was accomplished by nine local and international neonatal and maternal health stakeholders, researchers, and administrators. Respondents were asked to state whether all the variables and relationships in the CLDs existed and whether there were any missing significant causal factors. In case some elements were missing, they were asked to list them. Also, respondents tested whether the directions of each of the links were right or needed to be reversed (implying the effect is the cause) and were asked to state whether there were other effects could be observed as a result of the reasons in the CLDs.

Two CLDs emerged in next two figures depicting the factors associated with the supply and demand of health services for neonates and mothers. The CLDs were created from data collected from interviews in stage one of the study. Numerous reinforcing and balancing feedback loops can be observed.

The CLD dynamics involved in figure below identified frustration, lack of awareness, and trust, myths, and health support feedback loops. For example, the awareness is a virtuous cycle enhances not limits the growth of knowledge. The level of the neonatal and maternal health care improved the mother's health and confidence. Access to neonatal and maternal health services increased leading to lower risks neonate deaths. A mothers' preparedness such as improved awareness, family and community support, and socioeconomic status increased the likelihood of acquiring health services and having safer deliveries. The growth in the knowledge loop eventually slows down due to increased levels and interactions with health workers.

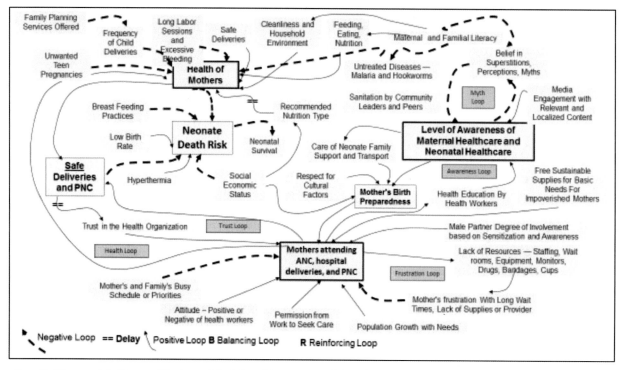

Part 3, Chapter 12, Figure 25: Agent Modeling Mapping Model and Systems Dynamics. Adapted by D. Anderson from Rwashana AS, Nakubulwa, Sarah, Nakakeeto-Kijjambu, Margaret, Adam, Taghreed Advancing The Application Of Systems Thinking In Health: Understanding The Dynamics Of Neonatal Mortality In Uganda. Health Research Policy and Systems. 2014;12(36):1478-4505

     The CLD dynamics in the figure below illustrates of the supply for neonatal and maternal health service presents a reinforcing or motivation loop representing positive workforce actions and balancing loops. These loops include transport, workforce, logistics, and workload. The loops reflect the desired goals towards improvement in the supply of maternal health services. The reinforcing and balancing feedback loops resulting from the systems dynamics was also examined. The potential high leverage points include individual gender considerations to ensure females receive essential education, thereby increasing maternal literacy rates and improving socioeconomic status enabled mothers to keep their infants healthy and more likely to utilize health services. Further, improved supervision and internal audits at the health facilities as well as addressing the gaps in resources (human, logistics, and drugs) facilitated sustainment of the program.[144]

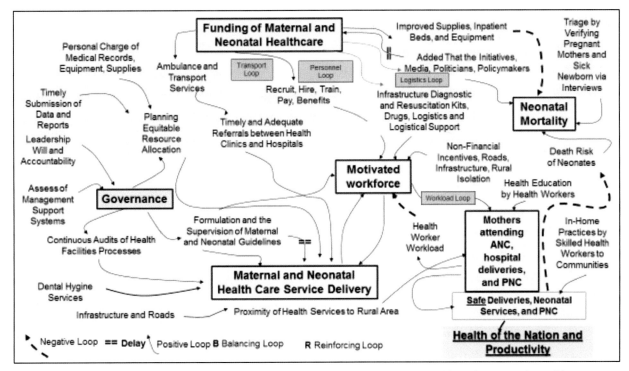

Part 3, Chapter 12, Figure 26: Use of Causal Loops Diagrams to Create Sustainable Solutions. Adapted by D. Anderson from Rwashana AS, Nakubulwa, Sarah, Nakakeeto-Kijjambu, Margaret, Adam, Taghreed Advancing The Application Of Systems Thinking In Health: Understanding The Dynamics Of Neonatal Mortality In Uganda. Health Research Policy and Systems. 2014;12(36):1478-4505

    Using CLDs facilitated deeper understanding and interpretation of the interactions and feedback loops contributing to the stagnant or dysfunctional neonatal mortality rates in Uganda. One of the key applications in this study was the inclusion of the perspectives of the different key stakeholders. These perspectives included those of the mothers, front-line health workers, and village health outreach workers. The findings suggest short- and long-term strategies using systems thinking could be applied in other settings to reduce the burden of neonatal mortality. For example, leverage, influences within the system where small changes (i.e., increased awareness and education, infrastructure support, and reprioritization of funding at the national level) can effect a substantial shift in the system was illustrated were underscored by the use of CLDs. Improved maternal and neonatal health service delivery will strengthen the virtuous cycle created by the motivation loops (i.e., motivated health workforce, acceptable workload). This effort represented a successful first step towards development and implementation of sustainable strategies to improve the health of the population in the short and term.[144]

PART IV: MOVING FORWARD

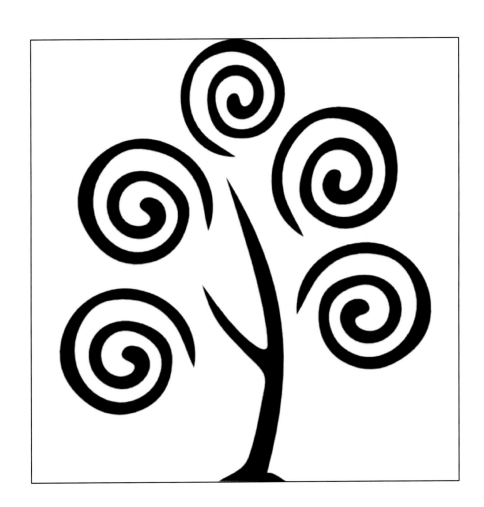

Summary of Part IV

Part IV provides a "thought leader" approach to the potential, possibilities, and aspirations of systems thinking to solve complex reoccurring problems and generate sustainable solutions. A variety of creative ways and means to implement systems thinking at the individual, team, organizational, community, global, and national levels exist. Each health leader must find what fits well within their organizational or community culture.

Global health leadership and leader development in the complex multi-stakeholder system will be a major challenge. Global health leaders at all levels must engage in big-picture thinking by developing the right set of competencies to quickly identify opportunities for sustainable change in a fragile and interconnected global health system. Health professionals are known for breaking patients down into a series of systems: skeletal, respiratory, digestive, reproductive, etc. and, in many respects, they are natural systems thinkers. However, health systems thinking competencies are not so widely distributed among leaders but much needed in a world of integration and interdependence. Health leaders will not only need to create a sustainable future, but they also need to curate the context by rethinking the commons and navigating through the paradox of letting go of linear thinking. Global health leaders must find and strengthen the vanguard for transforming "wholes" instead of parts. Global health leaders must create a culture of collaboration across organizations and system boundaries at all levels; engage in organized improvisation when opportunities emerge; and participate in global innovation sharing. Application of health systems thinking in a global health setting requires a more holistic approach to sustainable health development, health crisis response, and public health services.

Health leaders historically have been quick to satisfy patient needs in isolated ways such as cost, quality, and access. At the same time, many do not understand the systemic relationships with how community and community health systems contribute to poor health. Examples include increased costs, demand, disabilities, and disparities of care. Too often decisions are made simply based on the symptoms such as lack of access or long wait times. This long held pattern of behavior has developed over time and is a function of education, training, and experiences over many years. Health leaders must identify situations and opportunities where decisions can be made proactively. If health leaders look beyond the walls of their organization, understand the interrelationships of other systems within their organization, and collaborate with community health and non-health leaders in the context of the social determinants of health, innovative and sustainable solutions will lead to better health outcomes.

Like most other organizations, health organizations frequently find themselves stuck in balancing loops with less than desirable results; one example might be preventable deaths. Thinking and leading high reliability organizations in the context of systems dynamics and systems thinking will drive health leaders to break out of the fixes that have heretofore failed or achieved only limited results. To change the vicious loop of preventable harm requires a strategic and systems thinking mentality beginning with reframing the situation over time, looking for patterns and trends, and going below the surface of the pathological symptoms. These patterns are key indicators for the system and will enable you to determine leverage points will move the system to new loop results in desired outcomes.

Many challenges to implementing systems thinking exist with one of the biggest being traditional decision making and problem-solving habits. New forms of organization paradigms and leadership such as *Quantum Organizations*, as written by Ralph Kilmann, are emerging with a systems thinking component. Embedding health systems thinking into education and training programs is also imperative. Finding the balance between the present and creating the future has never been easy. For example, coming developments in transhumanism or the integration of person and machine interfaces with technologies such as artificial intelligence or prosthetics will require a profound understanding of the psychosocial, technological, and ethical aspects of this emerging trend. Integrating health systems thinking will go a long way in facilitating these growing phenomena.

Chapter 14: Need for Global Health Systems Leadership

Introflection

The competencies of global health leaders must include both strategic and systems thinking. As world health and non-health health leaders grapple with the future of global health, many common challenges and lessons will influence the future. As illustrated by the case studies in the previous chapter, the external and internal environments health organizations, health systems and societies operate in have become more fragile, as well as more interrelated and interdependent. This fragility will drive new and recurring problems and opportunities for health leaders. The possibility of catastrophic loss of life and impact on societies throughout the world such as disease outbreaks, communicable diseases (e.g. HIV/AIDS or Malaria), and non-communicable diseases (cardiovascular health and select cancers) is high. Areas, where significant investment in sustainable development has created gains, should be sustained, including promotion of women and children's health, building ownership and capacity, and generating global health innovations. Systems thinking considers the whole rather than individual elements and representation of the time-related behavior of systems rather than static "snapshots."[87]

Consequently, more often than not, actions taken to address complex problems lead to breakdowns is system functioning and failures of a program, initiative, policy or strategy, often creating feelings helplessness.[98,146] A reason for disappointing results tends to be the persistent focus on short rather than long-term thinking and underestimating the complexity of the problem or opportunity in question. As a result, most important sources of many problems are misunderstood, missed or overlooked and the decisions to eliminate them with quick fixes have unintended consequences that too often lead to undesirable outcomes, dysfunction, and policy resistance.[102]

Now, more than ever, health leader's must understand the fragile nature of health systems to find opportunities in chaos and understand how complex adaptive health systems throughout the world interact together. Navigating through the complexities and problems arising from the rapid pace of change associated with global health challenges and dilemmas requires health leaders to engage large quantities of information beyond their cognitive capabilities. Furthermore, health leaders must be able to sort through complex relations among parts of the system and keep pace with emerging opportunities.[87] Reducing adverse effects requires a holistic view of problems. Systems thinking competencies at the strategic and policy level is of paramount importance. It is critically important decision-makers understand and appreciate they are working within complex systems with interconnected and interdependent elements. Problems and opportunities should be approached as interactions among the system's elements versus focusing on single part incidents. This is the essence of systems thinking: the ability to see a global or community health system, not a single organization but as a complex system comprising many interconnected and interdependent parts and organizations.[87,97,101,49]

Help Wanted: Global Health Leader (GHL)

Health leadership, health leader development, and health policy development in the complex multi-actor and stakeholder system is a major challenge. Health leaders adept at systems and strategic thinking who are willing to suspend bias will seek sustainable solutions versus short-term or ill-conceived fixes that fail. Leaders will not only need to create a sustainable future; they need to curate the context by rethinking their commons or stovepipes and navigate through the paradox of letting go of linear thinking to see whole solutions. This action requires a particular kind of leadership: Global Health Leadership (GHL). GHLs must find and strengthen the vanguard for transforming "wholes" instead of parts and integrating the curative and preventive health systems at the community, region, national and international levels. Equally important, GHLs must create a culture of collaboration within and across organization and system boundaries. Thus systems thinking allows leaders to overcome the feeling of helplessness when confronted with complex problems. It gives them the necessary tools to inquire, analyze, understand, synthesize, and influence the functioning of the systems they are trying to improve. To begin the shift in leadership approaches, it is important to create a new approach to leadership that understands these concepts and characteristics of complex systems.

Regardless of setting or level, GHLs need to embrace systems thinking to navigate through the complexities inherent in today's health systems. Negotiating or getting to YES on sustainable solutions requires systems thinking, active listening, and negotiation as core competencies. Some of the biggest problems facing the world—war, hunger, poverty, and environmental degradation—are essentially system failures. For example, the Global Fund to Fight AIDS, Tuberculosis (TB), and Malaria, government organizations such as USAID and the Military Health System and non-government organizations such as Doctors without Borders, Partners in Health, and the World Health Organization, along with the Melinda and Bill Gates Foundation, can be proud of their global health accomplishments. These achievements are largely the result of vision, passion, and deeper understanding of the fragility and dynamic nature of the global health system coupled with a penchant to help through compassionate leadership. As the world becomes more chaotic, complex and interdependent, the need for global health systems thinking leadership becomes paramount to any future geopolitical landscape. Currently, there are many ongoing global health activities that are indicative of the interconnected world and overlapping stakeholder interests.[147]

Health systems thinking is a transformational and perhaps a "quantum way of thinking" that approches health systems development by integrating the social determinants of health with population health initiatives. For example, eradication of smallpox and treatment of diarrhea with oral rehydration solutions applied the principles of the social determinants of health was not a solution in isolation. The solution, using a systems approach considered the environment, population, patient, disease, project, or policy as a system. A fragmented and uncoordinated approach to sustainable development has too often resulted in unintended consequences such as dependency, inefficiencies, and inequities.[148] Therefore, the GHL's challenges cannot be solved in isolation or with a Newtonian (linear) approach. Even minor details, especially those associated with the social determinants of health have a tremendous ability to thwart the best efforts of linear thinking or the all too common political driven decisions.[41,47,148,149]

To accelerate transformation and innovative ideas to produce healthier communities and countries, more global health systems thinking leaders or GHLs are needed. This effort must include professional health administrators and planners, public health researchers and practitioners, and health professionals from all disciplines working together across traditional boundaries and communities to solve complex population health issues deeply embedded within the fabric of society. Avoiding a "tragedy of the commons" situation is important. The solutions will require simultaneous intervention and engagement with key actors, stakeholders and organizations across many levels ranging from local entities (i.e., schools, churches, work environments) to regional systems (health departments and hospital networks) to entire regions or countries (national agencies). This multi-level, multi-participant view is at the heart of systems thinking and GHL development, a developmental process of knowing how parts influence the whole local or global health system.[41,150,151]

Global Health Leadership Competencies

Today's global health professionals must possess the right set of competencies (e.g. a combination of knowledge, skills, and attributes) to succeed in a population-based health environment. If nations or communities continue to see the same issues or unsolved problems emerge over time, then it may be wise to reassess current competencies regarding their applicability and visibility. For example, the 2012 Institute of Medicine (IOM) report cited the annual number of preventable deaths in hospitals to be about the same as reported in 2001.[152] This repetitive situation represents a significant systemic problem. Also, the transition to accountable care organizations (ACOs) to deliver better health outcomes by improving coordination of health services with the local community health care system of systems will be required.[153] In many respects, the WHO and others face the same issues only on a grander scale.

Global health systems thinking competencies must be more pronounced in today's healthcare, educational, training, and leader development environments.[153] Systems thinking competencies offer the possibility of sustainable solutions. The expectations of the Sustainable Development Goals (SDGs), Healthy People 2020, and the Lancet Commission for Global Health 2030 require different ways of thinking about the chaos, complexity, and interdependence in achieving system-wide transformation and collaborative efforts. Public health experts assert systems thinking is aligned with ecological models, including epidemiological health, fragile human ecosystems, and the social determinants of health. Systems thinking today should not be the exclusive domain of public health leaders and medical social scientists, but should influence and infuse all health related disciplines.[154] The system thinking approach emphasizes how everything fits into the larger social, cultural, economic, and political system. The importance placed on interconnectedness cannot be underestimated in the 21st century. Incorporating systems thinking, system dynamics, emergence theory, and complexity theory as critical competencies would drive health professionals to view and solve problems of reliability, sustainability, and better health differently.[154] In other words, if sustainable solutions are to be produced in an interconnected and interdependent environment such as achieving SDG goals, reductionist approaches to improve health will be inadequate. Therefore, increasing systems thinking competencies throughout the leadership communities increases the ability to make sense of chaos, collaborate accordingly, and achieve SDG and HP2020 goals—ends, ways, and means.

Global health systems thinking skills are most applicable to the challenges faced by the global health and military health communities. Systems thinking is a much-needed discipline for seeing the whole systems or "forest for the trees" per se and identify and sustainable opportunities to improve. Connecting the political, economic, and informational systems to the public health and health system will provide the foundation for sustainable solutions. Further, systems thinking is a worldview, a process, and skill to better understand system's dynamics, generate sustainable solutions, and foresee patterns of change rather than static snapshots.[133] Understanding this aspect of health system development will drive leadership to invest in more preventive health and sanitary systems before making significant investments in brick and mortar hospitals and other facilities.

Behaviorally, global health systems thinkers must see both the pattern, behavior, interdependence of an event or challenge. This skill may require improvisation or techniques such as scenario analysis and back casting techniques. Systems thinking acknowledges strong or fragile interactions between system components, processes, and process owners to include emergent or unintended consequences resulting from interactions or induced changes. Positive system behavior change comes from an assessment of the interactions and following or assessing the relationships among the parts of a system. For example, before implementing a major health initiative, the need for a full logistics and security system analysis will help ensure future success at a reduced cost.[132]

Benefits

Collaborative efforts, especially fortifying the capacities of international health systems, are essential to prevent and prepare health security threats from natural or human-made infectious disease pandemics and chronic noncommunicable diseases.[155] Systems thinking leadership advances the rapid adoption of innovative solutions through inquiry, learning, and feedback systems.[24] Systems thinking is a process; an ordered, methodological approach to understanding problem situations and identifying sustainable solutions. For example, mobile health technologies are considered an innovative solution, however, understanding the underlying processes such as logistics support systems associated with implementing and maximizing the potential of mobile health is critical. This approach includes assessing the system within its environment or boundaries and the external context before actual implementation. Structurally, systems thinkers can see both generic and specific solutions, especially country or local population specific solutions.

While systems thinking is applied more prevalently in the public health settings, the application of systems thinking in other contexts or disciplines such as health administration and health policy is critically needed. For example, the World Health Organization (WHO) published a report titled *Systems Thinking for Health Systems Strengthening* in which they claim systems thinking is a paradigm shift. Public health is one part of the system. Systems thinking offers a comprehensive way of anticipating reactions, synergies, and mitigating negative emergent behaviors, with direct relevance for creating more sustainable system-ready policies. Systems thinking augments and enhances continuous quality improvement (CQI). As such, integration of multiple viewpoints is essential to systems thinking leadership. By having a solid understanding of a problem, situation, and environment, the systems thinker better understands stakeholder perspectives as a means to implement a global health initiative, policy, or process. As an imperative, the systems thinker must look at the problem in multiple ways through multiple lenses without reference to their bias. These insights or "ah ha" moments will result in sustainable solutions accepted by the stakeholders especially in a global health setting.[156,157]

By using systems thinking and understanding the complex interplay of the SDGs and social determinants of health and interrelated processes, the US and others will succeed in creating the ability to improve health and decrease the demand for unwarranted healthcare. Systems thinking will help health leaders and others achieve the vision of better health, improved experience of care, less cost per capita, and decreased morbidity and mortality; ultimately leading to a more prosperous nation. Health system leaders need to embrace systems thinking. Systems thinking has become a necessary competency for health professionals. By applying systems thinking principles and developing future health leaders whose core competency is systems thinking. Interconnections, relationships, and interdependencies affect health behaviors in the performance of policies and programs aimed at addressing key concerns. Leaders in the global and community health setting need to embrace systems thinking and learn to realize the many complexities inherent in a system-wide approach.[158] Complex systems thinking is a promising and potentially transformational way of looking at the world and our interactions with it. The concepts of complex systems thinking can greatly enhance our capacity to develop and sustain effective policies and programs.

Reflection

Systems thinking is both a worldview and a process; it can be used for both the development and understanding of a system and for the approach used to solve a problem. Health leaders, and practitioners must be more interested in ways to develop themselves as successful global health leaders. Health leaders need to assure organizations are structured to support a swift response to a crisis, create agreements, and actively engage winning the trust and confidence of international health partners. Leveraging and integrating health services builds relationships for human growth, economic development, and cultural diversity. GHL development supports international and national goals for eliminating dangerous diseases and helping develop sustainable, coordinated health system capacity among partner organizations and governments to prevent morbidity and mortality.

To be effective, health leaders must embrace GHL in the context of systems and strategic thinking as a necessary skill and responsibility. Systems thinking is the view systems, and problem situations cannot be addressed through reducing the systems to their parts. The uniqueness and behavior of the system are only present when the system is together—it is not a sum of the individual components. System behavior comes about as a result of the interactions and relationships amongst the parts. Also, systems thinking acknowledges the strong interactions between the system components, and the emergent behaviors and unintended consequences may result from these interactions.[25]

GHL offers health leaders an opportunity to increase positive perceptions and enhance the health of affected populations, greater security, and create mutual benefits for their organizations. Systems thinking contributes to this opportunity; as an ordered, methodical approach to understanding problem situations and identifying solutions to these problems. Systems thinking includes assessing the system within its environment, taking the external context into consideration. In systems thinking one sees and evaluates both the "forest and the trees."[132]

In the midst of complexity and confusion of many problem situations, systems thinking advances the understanding that solutions can be obtained through a deep learning process.[24,25] Health leaders can establish partnerships and exchange programs with international health counterparts to provide or train a cadre of medical and nursing personnel. Organizations with large groups of international patients can create customized health programs and invest in cultural awareness and sensitivity training to foster cohesion. Furthermore, improving responses to natural and human-made disasters, including complex humanitarian emergencies, ultimately benefits to entire global village.

Chapter 15: Integration of Systems Thinking with Strategic Planning

Introflection

Strategic planning and management are not a panacea for health organizations. Instead, strategic planning is a systematic approach to analyzing organization's situation (e.g. strengths, opportunities, aspirations, and desired results) and develop appropriate responses to achieve an aspirational vision with ends, ways, and means. One of the most useful tools for strategy analysis is systems thinking. To some leaders this sounds like a computer program, however, systems thinking is a way to think through big picture connections affecting an organization, strategic initiative, or policy.

Integration of Two Perspectives

Systems and strategic thinking have the potential to facilitate seeing the bigger picture and the interconnectedness of strategy formulation on health or public health system at the community, region or national level. This approach could come in the form of a scenario analysis such as impact (positive, negative, or opportunistic) of genetic screening, telehealth, mobile applications, and drones as tools for improving the health of an enrolled population at a reduced per capitate costs. The strategy is about forming an aspirational view of where the organization needs to be and how to get there. It is also about figuring how the right combination of ways, means, and ends with respect to implementation or strategy execution. A systems thinking approach to strategy has four stages and possibilities:

- Strength and opportunity analysis including understanding the systemic effects of alternative futures or scenarios
- Strategy development including various parts of the "as-is" and "to be system will behave to work together among new or revived parts
- Strategy implementation success depends on the amount of expected systems dynamics and the application of systems thinking tools to analyze complexity
- Strategy control and accountability alternatives such as empowerment, collaboration, and coordination across organizational boundaries and with partners

The strategic leader as a systems thinker will empower followers and stakeholders to be creative, share intelligence, and their wisdom to assure success for each of these stages of the strategy formulation process. The health systems thinking leaders encourages others to approach strategy development as a series of interrelationships rather than things or static processes, anticipate and see patterns of change rather than static snapshots. Combining systems thinking with strategy development results in increased creativity to generate ideas, analytic intelligence to evaluate ideas systemically, and generates the wisdom to balance the interests of stakeholders and ensure the actions of the leaders seek the common good rather than fixes that fail.

More specifically, strategy is a way to envision an aspirational or future state (ends). Systems thinking is about assessing the current or as-is state and developing sustainable plans on how to achieve the future state (ways and means). Both systems and strategic thinking challenge leaders to anticipate issues or find opportunities such as innovative new services or enhancement, adopt proactive, planning approaches to policy changes, and collaborate across organization and community boundaries to ensure healthier outcomes and greater experiences of care. Understanding the dynamics in the external and internal environment facilitates seeing patterns, behaviors, and trends, determining the best alternatives for resource allocation, assessing the implications and unintended consequences for creating value. As an example, an overall strategy to achieve better health at less cost could be converted into a strategic initiative such as becoming an accountable care organization (ACO) and improving the coordination of health services outside the walls of the hospital to avoid preadmission penalties.

Integrated with strategic planning, systems thinking is a way of seeing the world (i.e., "beyond the walls of the hospital") and how the parts of the system are related. Health services can be regarded as a "whole of a community" system of processes for delivering better health services (e.g. preadmission, admission, care and medication services, discharge, and follow-up through the episode of care). However, other subsystems such as partnering with hotels, home health agencies, transportation services, proactive patient engagement after discharge, and involving the family as caregivers "beyond the walls of the hospital" challenges leaders to think about the "system."

The benefits of adopting a systems thinking as part of strategy development are relevant in today's volatile, uncertain, complex and uncertain environment. Systems thinking allows leaders to counter volatility and uncertainty with vision and understanding such as ACO's bundled payment methods and readmission penalties as new paradigm of payment. Rather than isolate problems, systems thinking challenges leaders to reduce complexity by assessing the interrelationships, connections, and interdependencies before, during, and after a patient's discharge.

One of the cornerstones to any successful strategic planning process is organizational learning. Through learning, a shared vision and understanding can be articulated to engage support and participation. Learning, especially understanding the processes and interrelationships of entire system will minimize a tragedy of the commons situation. While quality improvement ensures the plan will use data in decision making, organizational learning helps foster adaptation to a changing environment. The skills of a strategic leader will need based on systems thinking since the organization is a complex adaptive social system. These skills and related competencies for different levels of staff, management, and leadership. The leader, as the chief strategist and systems thinker must think globally while considering the interdependence of managerial processes, leadership responsibilities, public health competencies, and the elements of strategy such as mission, vision, values, goals, and objectives. In fact, the strategic leader as the hub of a system of forces, influences, and responsibilities must act locally in order to assure system wide success. Today's health leaders must move beyond the walls of their organization to be successful leaders. In fact, these leaders would benefit from a public health leadership approach being involved with and remaining close to their communities, both internal and external. He provides a list of leadership practices can be adopted co help with public health leader sustainability.

Another consideration for the leader is organizational sustainability. This systems thinking mindset can be augmented by embracing a "triple bottom line." Instead of focusing only on the classic bottom line of finances, the leader connect financial viability, social responsibility, and the environment as part of the aspirational vision. By focusing on the triple bottom line and the application of systems thinking to strategic planning acceptance of the larger health system (thinking and living system) initiatives extending into the community second nature. To apply systems thinking successfully to strategy development, one must first define in general terms the preferred long-term outcomes or results. This mindset requires dialogue with the customer and supplier base. In healthcare or education settings, this refers to the entire populace. With the current information sharing capabilities of the nation, this is possible. To achieve a consensus on long-term outcomes requires explication of the consequences of decisions by the population.[20] This perspective, rooted in systems thinking, challenges health leaders to look beyond the walls of their organization for sustainable solutions in areas such as reducing infant mortality, ending homelessness, and solving the opioid crisis.

From a systems thinking perspective, this approach means the strategic planner or leader must develop a process for change management, not a structured, detailed strategic plan for the organization. It must involve relevant actors and stakeholders in the community as greater integration of the social determinants of health. Otherwise, the thinking, living, and open health system will reject static strategic plans. First, the system is composed of individuals who must collaborate across organizational boundaries. Second, they must be engaged and own the process or preservation of the status quo will prevail. Third, thinking systems self-organize, the parts co-evolve, and results emerge from these interactions. The triple bottom line guides leaders to achieve the ends in these objectives. If a strategist tries to implement a plan, the thinking system will still self-organize thereby changing the planning process; it will co-evolve by altering the initially designed structure and function. The results are unlikely to correspond to those originally intended.[20]

Changes will be necessary for leadership philosophy, worker culture, and the external environment. The interaction and interconnections of the health system parts must always be kept in mind. For example, governance structures of medical centers should include community health and non-health leadership. Public and community health and educational systems at all levels are not stovepipe organizations; they are interdependent and interrelated. For example, the solution to obesity is likely to be found at least partly in the educational process and vice-versa not in the treatment room.

School dropout rates will go down when children guided by their families and teachers learn personal responsibility for well-being and self-esteem.[20] They are needed to allow the system parts to interact rather than have conflicting incentives and contradictory values. This observation recognizes the system interacts with the external environment: these are open, not closed, systems. Accomplishing a change will require a champion with the strength of will to carry it out. Left to a strategic planning committee nothing substantive will happen.[20] A health leader focused on community-wide solutions adept at systems thinking will prevail.

Chapter 16: A Quadruple Aim: Integrated Community Health System Model

Introflection

For every complex problem a simple, neat, and straightforward solution always presents itself. Wrong! Health leaders and policymakers often think making a change in one part of a complex adaptive health system fixes the problem. Wrong again! Taking a systems approach to creating Integrated Community Health Systems (ICHS) would result in higher reliability healthcare delivery and healthier more productive population. Public health practitioners know the social determinants of health (SDOH) acknowledge the factors with the greatest impact on health outcomes are not medical interventions or lifestyle choices, but from the social and economic environments where individuals live, work and play.[125,159] It is time health executives and communities leaders do the same. Their focus is on community health and prevention. Similarly, effective health executives know a well-run hospital or health system has multiple service product lines, existing within even larger complex systems that must interact efficiently to achieve the best outcomes and experience of care for patients, families, and employees. This responsibility is otherwise known as the Triple Aim—better population health, best experience of care, and reduced cost per capita. Most successful health executives ensure attention is given to relatively small problems (such as near-miss events or under-staffed laboratory services) of a service and monitor the interdependent functions to produce the best possible outcomes. Community leaders or actors and stakeholders know their spheres of responsibility or influence affect the community as a whole in some large or small way. In many ways, these professionals are intuitive, natural systems thin inkers, however, the lack of collaboration and integration or a community-wide systems approach may be preventing these leaders of building a healthier community.[160]

Likewise, a person's health: curative or preventative is rooted in these complex systems of public, preventive, primary, and tertiary care, too. In most cases, it is well known the environment has the greatest impact on health outcomes across populations. But does the health executive wonder why there's so much demand, long wait times, or backlogs for health services (i.e., stock, flow, and rate issue)? Understanding this pressures and system dynamics requires a systems approach. For example, a child who is repeatedly admitted to the hospital with uncontrolled asthma despite medicine's best efforts. If a child has lived in poor housing with mildew everywhere or with roaches spreading asthma triggers for extended periods of time, medical interventions may not prevent the continual recurrence of the disease. In fact, building code standards, tenants' rights, and the availability of healthy and affordable housing have a direct impact the child's health. To effectively address asthma, non-medical issues must become a central focus of attention.[161] While this situation may fall outside the boundary of the healthcare executive, participation in alleviating poor health conditions should be. Unfortunately, medical and public health systems rarely or formally work together to form an integrated community health system (ICHS) unless there is a real opportunity (interest or incentive) or crisis. Asthma affects school attendance, which is directly related to educational achievement. Chronic absenteeism leads to lower education achievement.[162] This situation, in turn, has significant impacts on employability, wellness, resiliency.[163] Within the family, when a child is absent from school due to illness, a parent or guardian must care for the child. Parents risk unemployment if too much attention is spent on taking care of a sick child. This situation contributes to the affordability of health insurance and ability to bill for services rendered. Without basic prevention, the ripple effects of having a child who suffers from asthma could have impacts on family stability, training, and economic achievement. Without community leaders, actors, and stakeholders, the entire community suffers. This situation, in turn, creates more demand for health services thus creating backlog or medical appointment wait time challenges, a performance measure most healthcare executives are graded.[160]

Systems thinkers look for patterns of interaction among complex phenomena to better understand, analyze and articulate the current effectiveness of a system, and to diagnose how the system can be improved over time. Thinking about the challenges of Asthma provides an illustration on how integrating the principles of Triple Aim and integrating the SDOHs to improve health, wellness, resilience and community prosperity.[164] Systems thinking can provide the bridge between these groups to facilitate the development of a comprehensive approach to complex situations, opportunities, events or phenomena caused by isolated, independent, and usually unpredictable factors or thinking.[133] Systems thinking aimed at creating better health shifts the mind from seeing individual parts to seeing wholes or one's silo to seeing people and other organizations to active participants creating the future.[133] For health executives, systems thinking, in this case, lies in a shift of thinking to see interrelationships within the community rather than linear cause-effect chains of the backlogs and wait time challenges. Instead, health executives need to help design systems impacting community health and conditions as part of the episodes of care.

What is the Triple Aim?

The Triple Aim is a framework, illustrated in the figure, the Triple Aim was developed by the Institute for Healthcare Improvement (IHI) as an approach to optimizing health system performance. Health organizations must pursue three dimensions simultaneously: Improve the patient experience of care (including quality, safety, and satisfaction, improve population health, and reducing the per capita cost of health. In most health settings, no one is accountable for these dimensions. For the health of communities and patients, all three dimensions must be addressed. In addition to accountability for safe, reliable, and cost-effective care, the Triple Aim challenges leaders to harness the set of determinants of health, empower individuals and families, and substantially broaden the role and impact of primary care and other community-based services. By doing so, communities assure a seamless journey through the whole system of care throughout a person's life.[165,166]

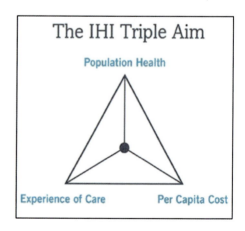

Adapted by D. Anderson

What are the Social Determinants of Health?

The World Health Organization states the "social determinants of health" reflect the conditions in which people are born, grow, live, work and age. Healthy People 2020 highlights the importance of addressing the social determinants of health as one of the overarching national population health goals of the current decade. The figure provides the visual of the SDOH.

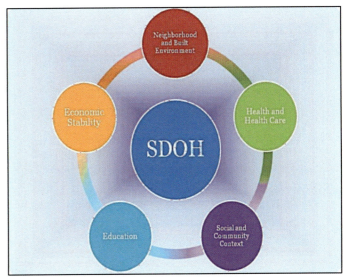

As the asthma case illustrates, the most basic conditions of life—quality of the family home, jobs with leave benefits to care for their sick children—have influences on health outcomes, not just on asthma but other preventable chronic health conditions. Leaders know having access to quality food, recreation, housing, transportation, public safety, education, and jobs are associated with how long individuals will live.[160] These aspects of family and neighborhood living conditions—beyond genetic inheritance and their poverty levels—have lasting health consequences.[159] When these essential aspects of civic life fail, a person is exposed to "toxic stress" which influences gene expression and brain development with direct and indirect adverse consequences for health.[159]

Quadruple Aim: Integrated Community Health System Model

Health organizations, insurers, and actuaries alone can only go so far with system integration and execution. Integration with public and community health, helping, and monitoring agencies are required to affect the health of the entire community.[165] It must work both ways too. Public health leaders and epidemiologists must collaborate to create a vision to develop an integrated community health system. It's reassuring when we see population health at the center of the model and national discussion. However, there is a communication problem here that needs to be acknowledged: what does "population health" in the Triple Aim model represent? The "population health" goal of the Triple Aim is the path to creating healthier communities by improving the experience of healthcare, especially patient safety and reduction of per capita costs needed for an integrated strategy. However, focusing on these two areas will not increase the health and prosperity of the community. The figure below provides a conceptual systems view of the Quadruple Aim: Integrated Community Health Model.

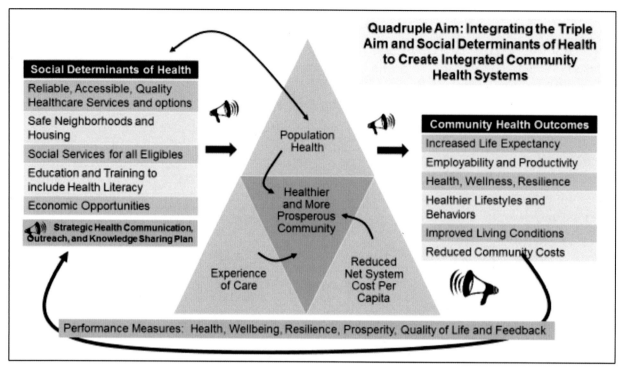

Part 4, Chapter 16, Figure 27: *The Quadruple Aim. Integrating the Triple Aim and Social Determinants of Health,* created by D. Anderson

As the figure shows, the SDOH relates to the population health and the desired health outcomes. This approach defines the relationship between community health outcomes (among populations, individuals, community services) how they are influenced by multiple SDOH. To achieve population health, the integration of the SDOH must be accomplished between all health and helping agency systems in the community.[167,168]

Health Leadership and Policy Perspective

To achieve the quadruple aim, effective population health management will require partnerships among providers, payers, and community helping agencies. Population health also includes integrated knowledge sharing systems and a focus on innovative patient or beneficiary touchpoints such as telehealth and mobile applications. Continuing the shift from fee-for-service delivery to community reimbursement models for the populations served will drive incentives aligned with better community health.[168] From a health policy perspective, research conducted by the Population Health Institute at the University of Wisconsin demonstrates that clinical medical care accounts for just 20% of health outcomes while health behaviors, socioeconomic factors and the physical environment account for the remaining 80% of health outcomes. Yet, only 3-4% of our national health budget is dedicated to disease prevention; the rest is dedicated to medical care delivery.[160]

This unbalanced distribution of the national health budget is illustrated by the fact the nation's largest single investment in prevention, the Prevention and Public Health Fund, provides $14.5 billion over the next 10 years,[160] while the total health care spending for 2014 alone was $3 trillion.[160] In short, communities are challenged to address the 80% of the causative factors for preventable disease with a fraction of the national budget on health. This imbalance is an impossible ratio bound to lead to failure unless something is done by challenging status quo.

The Triple Aim continues to be the gold standard for the transformation of the health system, linking improved experience of care, reducing per capita cost of care, and improving the health of populations. However, it should be linked to the social determinants in the form of the Quadruple Aim. Unfortunately, few health systems within and outside of the U.S. are incorporating the relevant tools and processes to address the social determinants of health in their systems of care. Without addressing and integrating the social determinants, improved health, wellness, resilience and community prosperity will not be realized.

Applying Systems Theory to the Triple Aim and Social Determinants of Health

By using an open and living systems approach to guide communities to identify positive or virtuous feedback loops, the smallest of changes in one discreet element of a complex system or personal paradigm can have multiple ripple effects on the other parts. While access to health care for individuals is necessary, community organizations must work at the systems level by taking a comprehensive approach to community health systems integration. Population health means doing business differently: integration of public health and traditional health care settings and other non-health or helping organizations. Integration of clinical, and community prevention services require aligning partnerships built for health, not just the treatment of symptoms associated with a disease. This approach will require community leaders, actors, and stakeholders to address social determinants with strategic partners not traditionally aligned with the health system. For example, socioeconomic factors such as poverty, homelessness, and education affect the prevalence of Asthma. If an asthmatic child often lives in a home with known asthma triggers such as mold, mildew, roaches, or second-hand smoke, there is little hope of preventing illness even if she has perfect adherence to treatment regimes. The Quadruple Aim can be used to challenge leaders to begin the dialogue and change perspectives to a more systemic understanding of this and other challenges.

Health leaders can no longer think of hospitals, labs, physician offices and clinics as the health system and their sole responsibility. Public health leaders must also be willing to venture into the population health system from a healthcare delivery perspective. The larger system should include housing, education, transportation, occupational health, and public health services. Addressing any number of public health challenges such as preventing chronic diseases, decreasing HIV/AIDS, opioid addiction, teen pregnancy rates, or increasing immunization rates globally requires a systems approach. Clinical Interventions may include telehealth, mobile health applications, and home health visits. All patients need screening, health education, and perhaps medication. Sometimes even the otherwise healthy and wealthy patients require hospitalization. For example, counseling and educational interventions help families and patients with asthma significantly reduce their health problems by knowing the event triggers and learning to manage symptoms earlier without inhalers and other medicines. Health delivery system leaders including actuaries and epidemiologists should work together to provide feedback loops in the form of knowledge sharing on asthma case trends and patterns of behavior.

Stakeholders such as hospitals, public health, and government agencies try to solve complex problems without engaging with and gaining the trust of members of the community most affected by systemic problems. For example, rather than seeing only isolated events followed by quick fixes (e.g., asthma, graduation, and employment rates), systems thinkers need to help leaders see the patterns of relationship (e.g., how unemployment is connected to higher school absences due to uncontrolled childhood asthma). When these patterns of relationship are projected over time, and historic data is used to make predictions for the future, the potential for sustainable solutions can begin to emerge.

With numerous stakeholders involved in a living community health system, complexity always lurks underneath with non-predictable adaptations to new circumstances. Health and public health organizations can support public policies, creatively leverage partnerships, engage residents on health and well-being of their neighborhoods, and implement preventive health education best practices to enhance community health. This action includes implementing and integrating recommendations (i.e., Tobacco Free Living, Preventing Drug Abuse and Excessive Alcohol Use, Healthy Eating, Active Living, Injury and Violence Free Living, Reproductive and Sexual Health, and Mental and Emotional Well-Being) across multiple settings to improve health and save lives. These actions also reduce the burden of the leading causes of preventable death and major illness.[169]

Seemingly isolated phenomena tend to be connected and influence each other over time. The challenge for the systems thinker, while embracing the unpredictable, is to find mutuality despite the diverse, divergent and stovepiped interests of those involved, as these key characteristics of a system emerge. Failure to address fundamental root causes may result in short-term "fixes" being inept and potentially harmful. If an action is taken without regard to how a short- term solution affects the entire system, long- term sustainable corrections will most assuredly be missed. Systems thinking urges stakeholders to focus on fundamental solutions rather than simply addressing short-term symptoms. Most health executives accept the responsibility of aligning all the functions of integrated hospital systems but have more difficulty dealing with domains beyond the hospital system itself for which they are not directly responsible. For example, achieving the Triple Aim includes assuring equity in access to care and driving out preventable diseases or living conditions contributing to disease thus leading to avoidable costs.

Reflection

Whether health leaders are working to understand how to deliver and pay for services for discrete or defined populations, collaborating with other health systems, or reaching out to the community to collaborate across sectors or SDOH on a community-wide health issue, the challenge will be greater integration and the leadership skill of systems thinking. Equally important, systems theory and systems dynamics offers useful insight into the dynamic and complex changes underway in communities. All community leaders are challenged to find patterns and related opportunities to address fundamental health conditions via the social determinants of health and the Triple Aim— avoiding preventable disease, unnecessary costs, and the drain on the health, wellness, and resilience of communities. This chapter provides an understanding of the need to integrate the Triple Aim and social determinants of health and challenges faced by leaders to create Integrated Community Health Systems (ICHS) leading to empower healthier and more productive populations. By applying a systems thinking approach long term sustainable solutions will emerge.

Chapter 17: Countering Pathological Archetypes to Improve High Reliability Healthcare

Introflection

Despite relentless and widespread efforts to improve the quality of health care in all settings, many patients still suffer preventable harm every day. Health organizations find continuous quality improvement initiatives difficult to sustain. They suffer from an inability to identify and counter the pathological effects of system dynamics and organizational fatigue. Problems thought to have been solved by one leadership team emerge in the form of a **Fix That Failed**. For example, a vice president of a large health system may choose to centralize training to meet budget cuts for a year only to find it three years later a new vice president of the same health system decentralizes educator positions to address unmet clinical orientation needs for newly hired staff. In health systems, the term complexity refers to a large number of coupled parts of a system interacting in countless in unpredictable ways. In many respects, health organizations represent the dynamic complex city where different effects and decision have consequences throughout the system. Although many decisions offer temporary relief such as the choice to centralize and decentralize training and education, the problem tends to resurface again creating a *"Tragedy of the Commons"* scenario. Systems thinking can serve to facilitate the development of sustainable solutions to achieve better health outcomes in the system including the community.

Health systems thinking refers to a set of interconnected and interdependent parts designed to achieve a particular purpose such as a health outcome. Today's health system is characterized by a complex of interdependent health organizations to advance and achieve a vision of healthier communities often produces the same harmful outcomes. It has been estimated 210,000 patients are harmed each year by medication errors in U.S. health organizations.[170] The importance of understanding the whole cannot be overstated. Systems thinking is part of the family of systems approach methods and tools offers an opportunity to eradicate the chronic diseases and pathologies or archetypes preventing health organizations from creating the most reliable organization in the world. For example, understanding and applying the thinking behind feedback loops may lead to a more mature quality management or systems approach to improving reliability in health organizations. Feedback about the quality of outcomes should guide efforts to improve the quality of the inputs and the conversion processes. However, in many cases, input, process, and outcomes are viewed as discrete and separate processes rather than the relationships and interactions among the parts.

High-Reliability Health Organizations

High-reliability organizations (HRO) organizations operate in complex, high-hazard domains for extended periods without serious accidents or catastrophic failures. Unfortunately, there are numerous examples of policy or change resistance contributing to the debilitating effects of unreliable healthcare. A study of adverse events in skilled nursing facilities (SNF) found 33% of Medicare beneficiaries discharged from hospitals to SNFs experienced an adverse event during their SNF stay. 59% of these events were preventable.[171] High-reliability science is the study of organizations in industries like commercial aviation and nuclear power operating under hazardous conditions while maintaining safety levels far better than health care organizations.[172] High-reliability in market-driven can relentless by the ability of health-related processes, procedure, or services to perform under common operating conditions as intended. Higher reliability should be attractive to health leaders due to the complexity of health operations and the risk of significant or potential catastrophic consequences when failures occur.[173] For example, the chance of a person dying from a catastrophic incident involving an amusement park, railway transportation, or aviation is less than one in 1 million. Healthcare organizations have been slow to embrace the magnitude of the failure to live up to an ethical imperative— deliver high-reliability care and adopt the techniques of high-reliability and a systems approach to doing no (preventable) harm.[174]

Several characteristics of high-reliability organizations are central to avoiding or minimizing harm in complex health delivery situations by creating a learning environment in practicing mindfulness or integrating strategy into the culture and standard practice. Unfortunately, many health professionals interpret high-reliability as standardization of health care processes. However, the principles of high-reliability go beyond standardization. High-reliability is better described as a cultural and social condition of persistent performance learning and mindfulness or being present – countering the pathology: eroding goals or drifting to low performance -- within an organization.[175] High-reliability organizations cultivate resilience by collecting, analyzing, and reporting patient safety-related information so continuous learning can be applied. Unfortunately, planning, designing, and leading integrated health systems is usually a patchwork of an individual, stovepipe technologies, processes, training, and user interfaces — seeking the wrong goal. For example, according to the findings of a survey and analysis of Baldrige Award recipients, high reliable care may be sacrificed –*Reinforcing A but Hoping for B* – at the expense of other competing goals.[176] The result is a constellation of technologies and perverse payment incentives to the detriment of patient safety, quality, and value or seeking the wrong goal. For example, at the patient level, different monitors emit competing alarms thus frustrating clinicians. Variation in medical supplies, equipment, devices, drugs, and billing practices generates frustration and drains mental energy. Increased documentation of care requirements causes delay or vicious feedback loops and diverts attention. Tense environments douse open communication creating missed opportunities for safe care, and –Vicious Reinforcing Loops—increasing risk, unreported near misses, unnecessary harm, and ultimately another preventable death. This situation leads to unnecessary patient harm, low productivity, excessive costs, and clinician burnout. Unfortunately, despite the past 20 years of the "Continuous Quality Improvement (CQI)" movement Drifting To Low Performance still plagues health organizations.[177]

Using Systems Thinking to Counter Harmful Patient Safety Outcomes

High-reliability organizations should systems thinking to evaluate and design for safety, but they are keenly aware that safety is an emergent, rather than a static, property. Countering negative archetypes – pathologies—requires a systems approach and collective mindfulness to place patients, families, and health teams at the center of an end-to-end process – before, during, and after the experience of care. To create collective mindfulness, the culture in a high-reliability organization stresses open communication among individuals, patients, and families at all levels.

The result is a High-reliability Organization (HRO) more aware of the dire consequences of even a small error or the ripple effect of overlooking these small errors.

New threats to safety continuously emerge, uncertainty is endemic, and no two patient events are exactly alike. Thus, high-reliability organizations serve to create environments where potential problems are anticipated, detected early, and virtually always respond early enough to prevent catastrophic consequences.[173] For example, integration of technology, people, and processes, so they are seamlessly joined in pursuit of a shared goal. An HRO approach may be new to health care, but the complexity and high-risk environments are not. For example, patient safety researchers at Johns Hopkins Medicine partnered with systems engineers and integrators of the Johns Hopkins University Applied Physics Laboratory (APL) as trusted agents to solve critical ICU challenges. The APL team guided patients, family members, clinicians, and researchers from many medical disciplines through a process of defining goals, understanding priorities, listing functions the system must perform, and determining measures of success.[177] These discussions led to reducing the common and preventable and social harms facing ICU patients. The team identified layers and layers of requirements for a system to achieve a shared goal—higher reliability. Through a combination of earlier warning alerts, common and transparent information, an environment of innovation, and culture of psychological safety resulted in less harm, better experience of care, and increased staff satisfaction.[177]

At the heart of creating an HRO, systems thinking enables many in health care to move beyond the "name, blame, and shame" approaches to improving reliability: focus on environmental, cultural and human factors engineering and the systems health care professionals can thrive in.[46] A systems approach to health reliability challenges health leaders to apply adaptive and innovative design methods to understand the whole or a system of interconnected components: people, machines, processes, and data to create planned, unplanned, and custom designed services beyond the walls of their organizations. The goal should be to focus on the outcome and *optimize*—rather than *maximize*—the performance of each of its components. Optimization is a value judgment by those who design, manage, and use the output of the system. And, stakeholders in the system, do not always agree on the relative priorities for the dimensions of the system's output.[174,178] For example, there is a growing movement to reduce readmissions, and Affordable Care Act (ACA) includes penalties for hospitals. They cost tens of billions of dollars throughout the health system. Now, hospitals are penalized with less reimbursement for readmissions – seeking the wrong goal. One in five Medicare patients are readmitted within 30 days, and one-third within 90 days, according to a *New England Journal of Medicine*. Medicare alone spends $17 billion on these round trips annually, and private insurers spend uncounted more dollars.[179] Increasingly, hospitals are realizing they can't manage post-acute care without help. A systems approach would challenge health leaders to approach the delivery of care from a whole systems perspective – inside and outside the walls of the hospital. No longer will a facility's responsibility for patients end when they roll out the front door at discharge -- working with patients and families upon discharge, learning about the patient's home situation, determining best options for care, and assigning a caregiver is slow to become the norm. Only through a systems thinking will this improve. While these initiatives are rarely reimbursed by Medicare or private insurance, the feedback loops should indicate the need to pay for them. For now, hospitals and nursing facilities absorb the cost – limits to growth.[180]

Systems Thinking and High-reliability Health Organizations at All Levels

More important, health systems are open living systems; that is, they are affected by—even dependent upon—larger systems of which they are a part and, in turn, they provide inputs to the larger systems.[174,175] In health care, the focus tends to be on microsystems. These microsystems are subsystems within macrosystems; the organizations such as hospitals, nursing homes, and clinics of which the microsystems are components. These incidents are part of the mega system of U.S. health care, which itself is a component of the even larger economic and social metasystems of American society as a whole. Complex systems and open systems are both at risk of producing unintended consequences, surprises, and opportunities. Even apparently "inconsequential" changes in health microsystems and health-related will almost always produce unintended consequences. While it is predictable unintended consequences will emerge, what those consequences will be—and whether they will be beneficial or deleterious—is often unpredictable.[174]

While systems thinking enables approaches to improve patient safety, it brings a set of unique challenges: unrecognized challenges impede progress and introduce more risk of patient harm. These challenges require health leaders to learn more about how to apply systems thinking to health care, through answering such questions as:

1. What are the microsystems and market-driven incentives in health care?
2. How can their performance be measured? Is there a feedback loop?
3. What are their vulnerabilities—and strengths?
4. What are the strengths and weaknesses of each component that comprises the system?
5. How can those strengths and weaknesses compensate for each other within the larger system?
6. How can the functions of each component be optimized so that the results of the system are maximized?
7. What are the interconnections and communications among the components?
8. How can health leaders identify and monitor unintended consequences?
9. How can health leaders intervene to prevent harm from unintended consequences?

The answers to these questions help health leaders frame the issues or opportunities to improve. For example, thinking in systems are mental models of the real world and how it works. No matter how close to complete and accurate our model may be, it is never entirely complete and quite accurate. And, no matter how useful this model is, it will never answer every relevant question health leaders can frame. That is why differing measurements of a system's components and outputs may lead to different or contradictory findings and conclusions. This situation is why different ways of analyzing these results can lead to various conclusions about how the system works or how it can be redesigned to make it safer.[174]

Reflection

By embracing and implementing a systems approach the potential to reduce patient harm improves. In doing so, health leaders must begin to rethink the design of health systems and the role of health teams—including physicians, nurses, and pharmacists—within the system. A systems-based understanding of how to prevent harm by countering organizational pathologies with learning and mindfulness will translate vision and strategy into common practice and culture. Adapting and applying the lessons of high-reliability organizations offer the promise of enabling hospitals to reach levels of quality and safety that are comparable to those of the best practices in other industries. An HRO mindset and further developments in transhumanism offer potential ways to counter pathologies and reoccurring problems in health organizations. A systems thinking approach has the potential and proven efficacy to accelerate the transformation of a health system from a riddled pathology driven system to one that promulgates higher reliability and much healthier populations.

Chapter 18: Epilogue – Leader Development to Think Globally and Act Locally

Call to Action

Now, more than ever, health leaders and policymakers at all levels must possess the right set of competencies (e.g. a combination of knowledge, skills, and attributes (KSA) to succeed in population-based health environments. The world, and especially its wide range of health systems, function in volatile, uncertain, complex, and ambiguous environment—a major challenge for health leaders and policy makers. Health systems are getting larger, more interconnected, and increasingly complex at every level. Each level interacts and impacts all levels. In many ways, we have to dance with or embrace the process, adapt to issues or opportunities as they unfold, anticipate surprise, and embrace that which emerges. Health leaders can't make the health systems conform to what they think is best. Health leaders have to give up being master decision maker and move willingly into an environment of ambiguity. Today, more than ever in this world, we need to be patient, expect failure, forgive one another, have compassion, and be present in the moment.[66][14,78]

Application of systems thinking to problems and strategy development in global, public, and community health settings is a way forward. Regardless of whether one believes in social or market driven national health reforms, systems thinking is called for. Perhaps in doing so we will find a "hybrid" or possible a third way. To fix world health problems, leaders are now compelled to recognize the interconnectedness of world health initiatives, events, and threats. For example, systems thinking methods and tools are increasingly being used to explain epidemics, syndemics, and to inform programmatic expansion efforts.[78] This fact requires nations and international institutions to address global health affairs differently.

Health leaders must apply the systems thinking tools to problems of community, regional, national, and global significance and, most importantly, work to effect sustainable solutions in the context public policy. In the future, quantum organizations and leadership will have finally traditional management extinct. Driven by quantum mechanics, quantum leadership will provide a systems-based model to provide skills for leaders to guide followers and partners others through unpredictable, non-linear and highly complex situations. This approach means generating innovation as close to the patient or customers as possible and managing virtual organizations and teams. At the personal levels, transhumanism will require a deeper understanding of systems thinking and system dynamics to improve the human factors associated with the person-machine interface and prevent the unintended consequences of poor decision-making related to development and implementation. For example, Transhumanism is an international and intellectual movement aimed at transforming the human condition by developing and making widely available sophisticated technologies to enhance human intellect and physiology significantly. Transhumanist and systems thinkers must study the potential benefits and dangers of emerging technologies that could overcome fundamental human, ethical, and limitations of utilizing technologies.

Systems Thinking as a Paramount Competency

If health leaders, regardless of setting, are continuing to see chronic issues or unsolved problems, then it may be wise to re-assess current competencies regarding their applicability and visibility. Systems thinking competencies offer the possibility of sustainable solutions. The expectations any health system reform requires different ways of thinking about the chaos, complexity, and interdependence of system-wide transformation and collaborative efforts. As stated throughout this book, the health environment has become more global, complicated, interconnected, and interdependent.

Increasing the popularity, availability, and applicability of systems thinking competencies offers a way to develop sustainable solutions and manage complex adaptive health system environments. Based on the discovery of detailed systems thinking competencies in public health and the increasing need to integrate the delivery of healthcare, population-based health programs, and community health systems, elevating the potential of systems thinking to other professional disciplines as a more prominent competency merits further investigation.

Systems thinking is particularly important for policy analysis, assessment of alternative policy options, and development of the desired right outcomes and measurement of those outcomes so learning and improvement can take place.[78] For example, the current system of measures, such 30-day survival thresholds after heart surgery and annual test scores for "No Child Left Behind", do not correspond to what health leaders think the public wants. To measure these outcomes requires long-term outcome measures. With such databases, educators could assess the best approaches to pre-school development, the optimal third-grade education program, and higher education choices. Without a database, leaders will face resistance and contradictory opinions and unintended consequences.[20]

Systems thinking approaches provide guidance on where to collect more data or to raise new questions and hypotheses. The methods and tools help leaders and policy makers make explicit assumptions, identify and test hypotheses, and calibrate models with real data. A more compelling reason to use systems thinking approaches is to inspire a scientific, unbiased habit of mind. Systems thinking can reinforce critical thinking, deep thinking either at the policy development or strategic management level. Systems thinking adds the new opportunities to understand, continuously innovate, test and revise creative solutions including how to intervene to improve people's health.[78]

Education and Training Community's Opportunity

Systems thinking competencies must be incorporated into education and training programs immediately. Systems thinking is a worldview, framework, and process for understanding a system's dynamics, seeing interrelationships, and generating sustainable solutions rather than static snapshots.[133] Systems thinking acknowledges strong interactions between system components and emergent unintended consequences resulting from these interactions. With positive system behavior change comes assessment of the interactions and relationships among the parts. Furthermore, systems thinking is a process; an ordered, methodological approach for understanding problem situations and identifying sustainable solutions. This process includes assessing the system within its environment or boundaries, and the external context. In the midst of chaotic problem situations, systems thinking advances the rapid adoption of solutions through learning or feedback systems.[24] Structurally, systems thinkers can see both generic and specific solutions. Behaviorally, they see both the pattern, interdependence, and the event.[132] In addition, multiple viewpoints are essential to systems thinking. To have a solid understanding of a problem situation, the health systems thinker must understand as many stakeholder perspectives as possible. It is imperative the systems thinker look at the problem situation in multiple ways and lenses. These insights result in solutions accepted by the stakeholders.[156,157]

As of now, many of the applications of systems thinking are derived from public and global health settings. This observation is the result of the nature of public health, adoption of systems thinking as a core competency, and embedded in many public health documents and texts. The World Health Organization's (WHO), publication on *Systems Thinking for Health Strengthening*, provides health leaders working in complex global health environments an overview of systems thinking, case studies, and principles.[16] However, the challenges facing all health organizations require a systems-based approach to generating sustainable solutions. While the American Public Health Association (APHA) has adopted systems thinking as a core competency and explained the core competency in detail (e.g. 12 statements), some associations have embraced systems thinking on a more limited basis. For example, a Health Leadership Alliance (HLA) study stated the competency database lacked attention in different competency areas. The HLA competency directory provided only a one-line summary of systems thinking in the context of change management and continuous improvement. The American College of Healthcare Executives (ACHE), competency assessment tool, includes only one line for systems thinking and no references, readings, programs, or self-study resources in their catalog while the Association of Nursing Executives (AONE) includes systems thinking and three statements on systems thinking principles. And recently, in 2017, the American Medical Association (AMA) in their Education Consortium released *Health Systems Science* to help guide medical education.

It is clear the health of any nation is a strategic imperative and at a deeper level, an existential requirement. By using systems thinking and understanding the complex interplay of the social determinants of health and interrelated processes, the nation will succeed in creating the ability to improve our health and decrease the demand for unwarranted healthcare. Systems thinking will help health leaders and others achieve the vision of better health, improved experience of care, less cost per capita, and decreased morbidity and mortality, ultimately leading to a more prosperous nation and world.

Systems thinking has the strong potential to transform how health leaders can shift perspectives to adapt and innovate, plan and lead, and grow and expand capacity for caring, for the living systems we are, relate to, and co-create.

Reflection

Today's health system transformation challenges require a new strategic and systems thinking mindset. Today's health problems at any level are rarely straightforward or unambiguous. Health executives and health professionals from all sectors and countries more than ever operate in the realm of bewildering uncertainty, staggering complexity, and increasing interdependence outside the hospital setting. These environments are often chaotic, complex, and interdependent. Elevating the systems thinking competency increases the ability to make sense of chaos and solve wicked health problems through of synthesis, analysis, and inquiry. In fact, systems thinking competencies need to be more pronounced in today's educational and leader development programs..

This book has presented a set of systems thinking concepts and principles, methods and tools, and applications including the need for health leaders to integrate multiple viewpoints or enhance strategic planning. In contrast to mechanical systems where individual parts interact to produce predictable outputs, complex systems interact nonlinearly over multiple parts and produce unexpected results or new opportunities.[112] Remember, the output of a mechanical system can't manipulate each of its parts, while the output of a complex adaptive system is dynamic, behaving differently according to its initial conditions and feedback loops. The broad range of concepts, characteristics and specific tools and methods presented with illustrative examples and vignettes in this primer should facilitate problem-solving and leader development. Sustainable health system transformation can only be achieved with creativity, innovation, and systems thinking. One of the opening statements of the American Medical Association 2017 publication, *Health Systems Science*, states, "Even if basic and clinical sciences are expertly learned and executed, without health systems science, physicians cannot realize their full potential on patients' health or on the population." Likewise, for leaders of health organizations, policy makers seeking health for all, and social scientists wanting a fuller understanding of health phenomena, these cannot occur without the informed embrace of systems thinking.

Appendix
Discussion Questions

Introduction: Systems thinking challenges health leaders to assess the interactions and interdependencies among elements (often competing) in a system, then seek out opportunities to generate sustainable solutions. The following questions explore the question of what and how systems thinking adds to the field of healthcare, public health, policy, and global health leadership. The questions are designed to help readers discover hidden assumptions, drive creative thinking, and express problems or ideas in a global manner. The questions are as follows:

Part I is organized in a way to provide a foundation (or refresher) for systems thinking utilizes levels of analysis from the micro (individual) to the meso (organizational) to the macro (global).

1. Systems thinking is an effective approach to help organizations, communities, and nations make sense of sometimes fragile interconnectedness and interdependencies of today's health systems. Why is systems thinking as a competency not sufficiently known nor embraced in health settings and across communities?
2. Integration of health systems at any level, suffers from reductionism and silo-like organizational models. How do the contributions of biology, ecology, chaos, and complexity theory contribute to characterizing the global health system as a complex adaptive system (CAS)?
3. Why is systems thinking important for health leaders at all levels? Summarize a situation or experience where systems thinking could have improved the outcome or success?

Part II provides an overview of concepts, methods, and tools for systems thinking with several illustrations and vignettes.

1. This primer introduces (or reintroduces) systems thinking as a promising approach to addressing today's and tomorrow's complex health challenges. The competency of health systems thinking marks a dramatic shift from the linear or reductionist and analytic way of thinking for several reasons Why is systems thinking hard to grasp and easy for others?
2. Given the health system's role in the health, wellness, resilience, and prosperity of a nation, evidence suggests a systems approach to improved integration, reliability, and health must be a priority. Summarize the terms systems dynamics, unintended consequences, interconnections, non-linearity, and sustainable solutions? Cite examples for each term.
3. Peter Senge created common archetypes or mental concepts as the most common set of patterns of behavior in organizations. Describe a real world dysfunctional archetype in your organization. How did it emerge? Why did it emerge? When was it discovered?
4. Find and summarize an example of a systems thinking tool or method that was applied in earnest to a stubborn or wicked problem and contributed to a sustainable outcome. What was the tool or method? How did it help participants discover possibilities and prevent organization dysfunction?

Part III reinforces the power of systems thinking with applications, and cases for health leaders, organizations, and policy in the public, private, and nonprofit sectors.

1. When health system and community leaders transform from an isolationist frame of reference to a systems thinking mindset, integrating multiple perspectives becomes obvious to understanding systemic problems and solutions. What does the term multiple perspectives or frames of reference in the context of systems thinking? Why is understanding multiple perspectives important?
2. Conduct a search to find a case study other than those summarized in Part III. Summarize the problem, degree of complexity within, outside, and between the organizations or groups, methods and tools applied, and the proposed solutions or outcomes. How could this case be applied in other situations?

Part IV challenges leaders and students about aspirations, potential, and possibilities of solving complex or wicked problems with systems thinking.

1. Strategic planning is a systematic approach to analyzing an organization's situation (e.g. strengths, opportunities, aspirations, and desired results) and develop appropriate responses to achieve an aspirational vision with ends, ways, and means. Whereas, systems thinking means the strategic planner or leader must develop a process for change management, not a structured, detailed strategic plan for the organization. How could systems thinking enhance strategic planning?
2. Today's health system transformation challenges require a new strategic and systems thinking mindset. Today's health problems at any level are rarely straightforward or unambiguous. Health executives and health professionals from all sectors and countries more than ever operate in the realm of bewildering uncertainty, staggering complexity, and increasing interdependence outside the hospital setting. They are chaotic, complex, and interdependent. Yet, curricula and courses on systems thinking is rarely found in healthcare, nursing, and medical education and training programs. Why? What do you recommend?

About the Authors

James A. Johnson, PhD, MPA, MSc

Dr. James A. Johnson is a medical social scientist and health policy analyst who specializes in organizational and systems development. He is a Full Professor in the School of Health Sciences at Central Michigan University where he teaches courses in comparative health systems, organizational behavior, and health systems thinking. Dr. Johnson is also a Visiting Professor at St. George's University in Grenada, West Indies and the former Chairman of the Department of Health Administration and Policy at the Medical University of South Carolina where he was also an Associate Professor of Family Medicine. He has been an active researcher and health science writer with over 100 journal articles and 18 books published. One recent book which is read worldwide, is titled, *Comparative Health Systems: Global Perspectives* where he and co-researchers analyzed the health systems of 20 different countries. The 2nd edition was published in 2018. He is also the co-author/editor with Leiyu Shi, Johns Hopkins University of the 3rd edition of *Public Health Administration: Principles for Population-Based Management*. Dr. Johnson is the past-editor of the American College of Healthcare Executives (ACHE) *Journal of Healthcare Management* and currently a Contributing Editor for the *Journal of Health and Human Services Administration*, and global health editor for the *Journal of Human Security and Resilience*.

He works closely with the World Health Organization (WHO) in Geneva, Switzerland and ProWorld Service Corps in Belize, Central America on international projects, often involving students. He is a regular delegate to the World Public Health Congress, most recently in Calcutta, India. His work and travels have taken him to over 45 countries so far. Dr. Johnson has been an invited lecturer at Oxford University (England); Beijing University (China); University of Dublin (Ireland); University of Colima (Mexico); St. George's University (Grenada) and University of Pretoria (South Africa), as well as, universities, associations, and health organizations within the U.S., including visiting or adjunct professorships at University of Michigan and Auburn University. Additionally, he has served on many boards including the Scientific Advisory Board of the National Diabetes Trust Foundation; Board of the Association of University Programs in Health Administration (AUPHA); Advisory Board of the Alliance for the Blind and Visually Impaired; Board President of Charleston Lowcountry AIDS Services; Advisory Board of the Joint Africa Working Group; Board of Directors of the Africa Research and Development Center; Advisory Board of the Center for Collaborative Health Leadership; Board of Advisors for Health Systems of America; and a member of the Governing Council of the American Public Health Association (APHA). Dr. Johnson completed his Ph.D. at Florida State University where he specialized in health policy and organization development. He also has a M.P.A. in health care administration and policy from Auburn University and a M.Sc. in behavioral science.

Douglas E. Anderson, DHA, MSS, MBA, FACHE

Dr. Douglas E. Anderson is a former Colonel in the Air Force (AF) Medical Service Corps (MSC) with 30+ years of experience: leadership, strategic management, quality improvement, policy development, and education experiences. He completed a Doctor of Health Administration (DHA) degree and certificate in International Health at Central Michigan University (CMU). His dissertation on Strategic Health Enterprise Leaders illustrates why development of future strategic-minded health leaders are needed to create the world' most reliable and innovative health system and healthiest population.

He's been a successful corporate staff officer, CEO, and COO at multiple health facilities leading high performance teams or implementing system-wide initiatives. He acquired strategy development, program management, and leadership experience in multiple departments, levels and career broadening assignments. He has served as a strategist, strategic communicator, CIO, CFO, and disaster preparedness officer at the multi-health system, joint, or service-level corporate staff levels. Prior to earning his DHA, he served directly for the Air Force Surgeon General (SG) as the Director of Strategic Health Communication and Organizational Improvement. He completed a 1-year tour in Afghanistan as the senior advisor and team lead to the Afghanistan National (ANP) SG to help build his health system and train corporate headquarters staffs on health delivery. As CEO, he led a 400-person 42 provider medical group practice serving 72,000 beneficiaries with a volume of 141,000 annual visits on a $46,000,000 budget. He spent four years at the Air Force Office of Homeland Security and Joint Forces Command as a health strategist and health planner to create "joint" policies and futures concepts. He also served as the Joint Task Force Surgeon's course director.

He currently serves as an adjunct faculty member and healthcare consultant. He's developed a federal health merger evaluation plan, conducted leader development training, and served as a federal health futurist, event planner, and facilitator. He's developed and delivered numerous educational programs and presentations on managing health organizations, strategy and change management, leader development, quality improvement, strategic communication, and global health engagement. He developed six new master of health administration courses. He recently delivered a 3-hour seminar on preparing for strategic health leadership at the 2017 American College of Healthcare Executives (ACHE) conference.

As a lifelong learner, he earned master's degrees in Military Strategic Studies (MSS) from Air University, Master of Business Administration (MBA) from University of Central Missouri, and a Master of Arts (MA) from CMU. He is Fellow in the American College of Healthcare Executives (ACHE). He currently serves as Vice President of the Air Force MSC Association, member, Air Force Association Veteran's Council and member of the West Virginia Panhandle Building Healthier Communities Cooperative.

References

1. Waldman D. We can fix healthcare: Thinking Systems Need Systems Thinking. 2007. http://www.wecanfixhealthcare.info/thinking-systems-need-systems-thinking.html.
2. Kauffman Dl, Jr.,. *Systems One: an Introduction to Systems Thinking.* Minneapolis, Minnesota: Future systems Inc., S. A. Carlton; 1980.
3. Govette J. This INSANE Graphic Shows How Ludicrously Broken the Healthcare Referral System Really Is. *ReferralMD*. San Fransisco: ReferralMD; 2013.
4. Hostetter M, Klein, Sarah. Hospitals Invest in Building Stronger, Healthier Communities. *Transforming Care.* 2016. http://www.commonwealthfund.org/publications/newsletters/transforming-care/2016/september/in-focus.
5. Shortell SM GR, Anderson DA, Mitchell JB, Morgan KL. Creating organized delivery systems: The barriers and facilitators." *Hospital & Health Services Administration* 1993;38(4):447-466.
6. Fadul R. The Tragedy of the Commons Revisited. *N Engl J Med* 2009;361(10):1055.
7. Mercola J. Top Ten Ways the American Health Care System Fails. Paper presented at: Mayo Clinic Proceedings2014; Harper College, MN.
8. Califf RM. 21st Century Cures Act: Making Progress on Shared Goals for Patients. In: Voice F, ed. *US Government*. Washington DC: Food and Drug Administration (FDA); 2016.
9. Kauffman D, Jr. *Systems One: Introduction to Systems Thinking by Future Systems, The Innovative Learning Series.* Minneapolis, MN, USA: S.A. Carlton; 1980.
10. Klien E. Ten Reasons Why American Health Care Is so Bad. *The Amercian Prospect.* Washington DC: Washington Post; 2007.
11. n.a. Seeking the Wrong Goal. *Systems & Us: Embracing Complexity*
12. Mattke S, Hangsheng Liu, Emily Hoch and Andrew W. Mulcahy. *Avoiding the Tragedy of the Commons in Health Care: Policy Options for Covering High-Cost Cures.* Santa Monica, CA: RAND Corporation;2016.
13. Stroh D. *Systems Thinking For Social Change: A Practical Guide to Solving Complex Problems, Avoiding Unintended Consequences, and Achieving Lasting Results.* 85 N Main St, #120, White River Junction, VT 05001-7059: Chelsea Green Publishing; 2015.
14. Wheatley M, J. *Leadership in the New Science: Discovering Order in a Chaotic World.* San Francisco, California: Berrett – Koehler publishers Inc.; 1999.
15. Johnson J, Rossow, C. *Health Organizations: Theory, Behavior, and Development. .* Burlington, MA: Jones and Bartlett (J&B); 2018.
16. Savigny Dd, Adam, Taghreed. *Systems Thinking for Health Systems Strengthening.* Geneva, Switzerland: World Health Organization (WHO);2009.
17. Johnson JA, Stoskof, Carleen H. *Comparative Health Systems: Global Perspectives.* Sudbury, MA, USA: Jones and Bartlett, LLC; 2010.
18. Hirsch ED, Kett, Joseph F., Trefil, James S. *Cultural Literacy: What Every American Needs to Know.* Vancouver, Canada: Vintage Books; 1988.
19. Algoso D. Zooming out from healthcare to systems thinking. 2014. http://algoso.org/2014/04/06/zooming-out-from-healthcare-to-systems-thinking/.
20. Waldman D. Systems Thinking and…The U.S. Healthcare System. *Triarchy Press*2008.
21. Donovan T, Kenneth, Hoover *The Elements of Social Scientific Thinking, 2nd Edition.* Boston, MA: Cengage Learning; 2013.

22. Heylighen F. Basic Concepts of the Systems Approach. 1998. http://www.pespmc1.vub.ac.be/SYSAPPR.html.
23. Heylighen F, Joslyn, C. What is Systems Theory? . 1992. http://www.pespmc1.vub.ac.be/SYSTHEOR.html.
24. Checkland P. *Systems Thinking, Systems Practice.* New York: John Wiley & Sons; 1999.
25. Krieger L. Systems Thinking Simplified. 2000.
26. Von Bertalanffy L. *General Systems Theory.* New York: George Braziller; 1968.
27. Goldstein J. *Conceptual Foundations of Complexity Science: Development and Main Concepts.* Charlotte, North Carolina: Information Age; 2008.
28. Jung DI, Chow, C., & Wu, A. The Role of Transformational Leadership in Enhancing Organizational Innovation: Hypotheses and Some Preliminary Findings. *The Leadership Quarterly.* 2003;14 525-544.
29. Lord R. Beyond Transactional and Transformational Leadership: Can Leaders Still Lead When They Don't Know What to Do? In: Marion MU-BR, ed. *Complexity Leadership Part One: Conceptual Foundations.* Charlotte, NC: Information Age Publishing; 2008:155-184.
30. Ibarra H, Kilduff, M., Tsai, W. Zooming in and out: Connecting Individuals and Collectivities at the Frontiers of Organizational Network Research. *Organization Science.* 2005;16(4):359 – 371.
31. Plowman DA, & Duchon, D. *Dispelling the Myths about Leadership: from Cybernetics to Emergence.* Charlotte, NC: Information Age Publishing.: Information Age Publishing; 2008.
32. McKelvey B. Emergent strategy via complexity leadership: Using complexity science and adaptive tension to build distributed intelligence. In: Marion MU-BR, ed. *Complexity leadership part 1: Conceptual foundations* Charlotte, NC: Information Age; 2008 225-268.
33. Uhl-Bien M, Marion, R. *Complexity leadership part 1: Conceptual foundations.* Charlotte, NC: Information Age Publishing.; 2008a.
34. Heylighen FJ, C.; Turchin, V. What are Cybernetics and Systems Science? . 1993. http://www.pespmc1.vub.ac.be.CYBSWHAT.html.
35. Reid PP, Compton, W. Dale, Grossman, Jerome H., Fanjiang, Gary. *Building a Better Delivery System: A New Engineering/Health Care Partnership.* Washington DC: National Academies of Press (NAP); 2005.
36. Bellinger G. Systems Thinking: an Operational Perspective of the Universe. *Outsights.* 1998.
37. Bruner J. *Going Beyond the Information Given.* New York: Norton; 1974.
38. Lipsitz LA. Understanding Health Care as a Complex System, The Foundation for Unintended Consequences. *JAMA.* 2012;308(3):243-244.
39. Anderson DE. Call to Action: Identifying the Need To Apply Systems Thinking Competencies In the Healthcare Setting. Mount Pleasant, Michigan: Central Michigan University, Doctorate of Health Administration Program; 2013.
40. Firesen M, Johnson, James A. The Success Paradigm: Creating Organizational Effectiveness Through Quality and Strategy. Seattle, Washington: Amazon Digital Services LLC 1995.
41. Campbell S. *Flagship Report: Systems Thinking for Health Systems Strengthening.* Alliance for Health Policy and Systems Research; 2009.

42. Quinn JB. *Intelligent Enterprise: A Knowledge and Service Based Paradigm for Industry.* New York: Free Press; 1992.
43. Nelson EC, P.B. Batalden, J.J. Mohr, and S.K. Plume. Building a quality future. *Frontiers of Health Services Management* 1998;15(1):3-32.
44. Ferlie EB, and S.M. Shortell. Improving the quality of health care in the United Kingdom and the United States: a framework for change. *Milbank Quarterly.* 2001;79(2):281-315.
45. McGlynn EA, S.M. Asch, J. Adams, J. Keesey, J. Hicks, A. DeCristofaro, and E.A. Ker. The quality of health care delivered to adults in the United States. . *New England Journal of Medicine.* 2003;348(26):2635-2645.
46. ST4CHealth. An Introduction to Complex Systems Thinking in Health. 2016; https://st4chealth.com/.
47. Beaglehole R, Bonita, Ruth. What is Global Health? *Global Health Action.* 2010; 3(10):3402.
48. Koplan JPea. Towards a common definition of global health. *The Lancet.* 2009;373(9679):1993–1995.
49. Lebcir RM. Health Care Management: The Contribution of Systems Thinking. Management Systems Department The Business School: University of Hertfordshire College Lane, Hatfield, Herts AL10 9AB, UK; 2006.
50. Ledlow GaNC, and Jones & Bartlett Learning, LLC. Leadership for Health Professionals, Chapter 16 - Leadership System Template. 2010. https://docs.google.com/viewer?a=v&q=cache:_FkOFhKCwzUJ:samples.jbpub.com/9780763781514/81514_CH16_LeadershipSystemTemplate.doc+&hl=en&gl=us&pid=bl&srcid=ADGEESivsaKXDhQJE7nYrRGo8HB0btDDa48RSBd-1t5acznWf6jkbqxPbyhsqPc8itv5LjwrR9q-0Yi4F-ma-gKrSXkIMct5U85RA.
51. Masterson B, Calvo, Ahmed, Jonas, Wayne Creating the Future of Health: The Journey. In: Masterson B, ed. *Health Futures Group (HFG).* Washington DC: National Defense University (NDU); 2013a.
52. Rubino L, Esparza, Salvador, Chassiakos, Yolanda. *New leadership for today's healthcare professionals: concepts and cases.* Burlington, Massachusetts,: Jones and Bartlett Learning; 2014.
53. Cosgrove D, Fisher, M., Gabow, P., Gottlieb, G., Halverson, G. *A CEO checklist for high value healthcare.* Washington DC: Institute of Medicine of the national academies; 2012.
54. Nickerson J, Sanders, Ronald. *Tackling Wicked Government Problems: A Practical Guide for Developing Enterprise Leaders.* Washington DC: Brookings Institute Press; 2013.
55. Sanders TI. *Strategic thinking and the new science: Planning in the midst of chaos, complexity, and change.* New York, NY: The Free Press; 1998.
56. Masterson B, Moore, Frank, Rosenkrans, Wayne. Organizational Agility: A Framework for Facilitating Transformation. In: Masterson B, ed. *Health Futures Group (HFG).* Washington DC: National Defense University (NDU); 2013c.
57. Chatterjee A KS, King J, DeVol R. *Checkup Time: Chronic Disease and Wellness in America.* Milken Institute; 2014.
58. Stewart WF, Ricci, Judith A., Chee, Elsbeth, Morganstein, David. Lost Productive Work Time Costs From Health Conditions in the United States: Results From the American Productivity Audit. *Journal of Occupational and Environmental Medicine (JOEM).* 2003;45(12):1234-1236.

59. Shreve J, Van Den Bos, Jill, Gray, Travis, Halford, Michael. Rustagi, Karan, Ziemkiewicz, Eva *The Economic Measurement of Medical Errors.* Milliman, Inc.; 2010.
60. Musgrove P, "The World Health Report 2000, Health Systems: Improving Performance," World Health Organization, http://www.who.int/whr/2000/en/whr00_en.pdf *The World Health Report 2000, Health Systems: Improving Performance.* World Health Organization (WHO); 2000.
61. NRC. *U.S. Health in International Perspective: Shorter Lives, Poorer Health.* . Washington, DC: The National Academies Press; 2013.
62. Fuchs V. Challenges in Health Care Costs New York, New York: New York Times; 2012.
63. IOM. *Crossing the quality chat zone: a new health system for the 21st century.* Washington DC: National Academy Press;2001.
64. Kohn. L.T. C, J.M., . *To Err Is Human: Building a Safer Health System.* Washington, DC: Institute of Medicine (IOM);1999,.
65. Masterson B, Sanders, Ron. *DOD GLOBAL HEALTH ENGAGEMENT ALTERNATIVE FUTURES [NIGERIA-EBOLA] SCENARIO WORKSHOP SUMMARY OUTBRIEF.* National Defense University (NDU);2014.
66. Wheatley M, J. *Leadership in the New Science: Learning about Organization from an Orderly Universe.* San Francisco, California: Berrett – Koehler publishers Inc.; 1992.
67. Edson R. *Systems Thinking. Applied. Version 1.1.* ANSER Corporation, ASyst Institute; 2008.
68. Liu P, Wu, Shinyi. *Health Care Management Science.* 2016;19:89-101.
69. Bae S-H, Nikolaev, Alexander, Seo, Jin Young, Castner, Jessica Castner. Health care provider social network analysis: A systematic review. *Nursing Outlook.* 2015;63, Issue 5, Pages 566–584 (5):566–584
70. DR E, NJ, Beauchamp, A., Norbash. Scenario planning. *Journal of the American College Radiology.* 2011;;8(3):(3):175-179. doi: .
71. Homer J, Jones, Andrew, Seville, Don, Essien, Joyce, Milstein, Bobby, Murphy, Dana The CDC's Diabetes Systems Modeling Project: Developing a New Tool for Chronic Disease Prevention and Control 22nd International Conference of the System Dynamics Society 2004; Oxford, England.
72. n.a. Health and Disease. 2016; https://steps-centre.org/health-disease/.
73. Tsan A, Sheng, Tsan Sheng, Sy, Charlle, Li, Jie. A SYSTEM DYNAMICS MODEL OF SINGAPORE HEALTHCARE AFFORDABILITY. Paper presented at: Winter Simulation Conference2011; Singapore.
74. Branscomb J. *Systems Thinking Tools and Principles for Collaboration and Problem Solving.* Georgia Health Policy Center, Atlanta, Georgia: Healthcare Georgia Foundation;2016.
75. Colligan L, Anderson, Janet E., Potts, Henry WW, Berman, Jonathan. Does the process map influence the outcome of quality improvement work? A comparison of a sequential flow diagram and a hierarchical task analysis diagram. *BMC Health Serv Res* 2010;10(6).
76. Gillies A, Maliapen, Mahendran Using healthcare system archetypes to help hospitals become learning organisations. *Journal of Modelling in Management.* 2006;3(1):82-99.
77. Bishai D, Paina, L, Li, Q, Peters, DH, Hyder, A. Advancing the application of systems thinking in health: why cure crowds out prevention. *Health Res Policy Syst* 2014;12:12-18.

78. Peters DH. The Application of Systems Thinking in Health: Why Use Systems Thinking? *Health Research Policy and Systems* 2014;12(51).
79. Luke DA H, JK. Network analysis in public health: history, methods, and applications. *Annu Rev Public Health.* 2007;28:69-93.
80. Malik A, Willis, CD, Hamid S, Ulikpan A, Hill, PS. Advancing the application of systems thinking in health: advice seeking behavior among primary health care physicians in Pakistan. *Health Res Policy Syst* 2014;12:43.
81. Goulet H, Guerand, Victor, Bloom, Benjamin, Martel, Patricia, Aegerter, Philippe, Casalino, Enrique, Riou, Bruno, Freund, Yonathan Unexpected death within 72 hours of emergency department visit: were those deaths preventable? *Critical Care.* 2015;19:154.
82. Zhang X, Bloom, G, Xu, X, Chen, L, Liang, X, Wolcott, SJ. J: Advancing the application of systems thinking in health: managing rural China health system development in complex and dynamic contexts. *Health Res Policy Syst.* 2014;12:44.
83. McKenzie A, Abdulwahab, Ahmad, Sokpo, Emmanuel, Mecaskey, Jeffrey W. . *Building a Resilient Health System: Lessons from Northern Nigeria.* Brighton, BN1, 9RE, UK Institute of Development Studies;2015.
84. Epstein J. Why model? *J Artif Soc Soc Simulat.* 2008;11(4):12.
85. Anderson V, Johnson, Lauren. *Systems Thinking Basics: from Concepts to Causal Loops.* First edition ed. Westford, Massachusetts: Pegasus Communications, Inc.; 1997.
86. Meadows D, H. *Thinking and Systems: a Primer.* White River Junction, Vermont: Chelsea Green Publishing; 2008.
87. Senge PM. *The Fifth Discipline: The Art & Practice of the Learning Organization. .* New York: Doubleday/Currency; 1990.
88. n.a. *Bridging the Evidence Gap in Obesity Prevention: A Framework to Inform Decision Making.* Washington, DC: U.S. Institute of Medicine (IOM);2010.
89. Hamid TKA. *Thinking in Circles About Obesity: Applying Systems Thinking to Weight Management).* Gewerbestrasse 11, CH-6330 Cham (ZG), Switzerland: Springer International Publishing; 2009.
90. Kumanyika SK, Parker, Lynn, Sim, Leslie J. *Bridging the Evidence Gap in Obesity Prevention: A Framework to Inform Decision Making.* Washington DC: National Academies of Press (NAP); 2010.
91. Frood S, Johnston, Lee M., Matteson, Johnston, Carrie L., Finegood, Diane T. Obesity, Complexity, and the Role of the Health System. *Curr Obes Rep.* 2013; 2(4):320-326.
92. Hamid TKA. Thinking in Circles About Obesity. *Systems Thinker.* 2009. https://thesystemsthinker.com/thinking-in-circles-about-obesity/.
93. Muraven M, Tice, DM, Baumeister, R. F. Self-control as a limited resource: Regulatory depletion patterns. *Journal of Personality and Social Psychology.* 1998;74.
94. Meadows DH. *Thinking in Systems, A Primer.* White River Junction, VT, USA: Chelsea Green Publishing Company; 2008.
95. M. Muraven DMT, and R. F. Baumeister. Self-control as a limited resource: Regulatory depletion patterns. *Journal of Personality and Social Psychology.* 1998;74.
96. Finegood D. The importance of systems thinking to address obesity. *Nestle Nutr Inst Workshop Ser* 2012;73:123-137.
97. Forrester J. *Industrial dynamics.* Cambridge, MA: The MIT Press 1961.
98. Sterman J. *Business Dynamics: Systems Thinking and Modeling for a Complex World.* Boston, Massachusetts: Irwin McGraw-Hill.; 2000.

99. WHO. Health promotion glossary. World Health Organization 1998.
100. Milstein B. Overview of System Dynamics Simulation Modeling. Systems Thinking and Modeling Workshop; 2006; Bethesda, MD.
101. Sterman J. System Dynamics modelling: tools for learning in a complex world. *California Management Review.* 2001;43(4):8-25.
102. Sterman J. Learning in and about complex systems. *System Dynamics Review.* 1994;10(2-3):291-330.
103. Sengupta K, Abdelhamid TK. Coping with staffing delays in software project management: An experimental Investigation *Management Science.* 1993;39(4):411-428.
104. Sengupta K AT, and Bosley M. Coping with staffing delays in software project management: An experimental Investigation. *IEEE Transactions on systems, Man, and Cybernetics, Part A,.* 1999;29(1):77-91.
105. Plsek P. *Redesigning health care with insights from the science of complex adap tive systems. In: Crossing the Quality Chasm: A New Health System for the 21st Century.* Washington DC: The National Academies Press;2001.
106. Sturmberg JP OHD, Martin CM. Understanding health system reform—a complex adaptive systems perspective. *J Eval Clin Pract.* 2012;18(1): 202-208.
107. Congress U. H.R.6 - 21st Century Cures Act. In: Means H-EaCWa, ed. Washington DC: Senate - Health, Education, Labor, and Pensions; 2016.
108. Jha AK JK, Orav EJ, Epstein AM. The long-term effect of premier pay for performance on patient outcomes. *N Engl J Med.* 2012;366(17):1606- 1615.
109. Nelson L. *Lessons from Medicare's demonstration projects on disease man- agement, care coordination, and value-based payment; 2012.* Washington, DC: Congressional Budget Office; 2012.
110. Shackelton RJ ML, Link CL, McKinlay JB. The intended and unintended consequences of clinical guidelines. *J Eval Clin Pract.* 2009;15(6):1035- 1042.
111. Boyd CM DJ, Boult C, Fried LP, Boult L, Wu AW. Clinical practice guide- lines and quality of care for older patients with multiple comorbid diseases: implications for pay for performance. *JAMA.* 2005;294(6):716-724.
112. Lipsitz LA. Understanding Health Care as a Complex System: The Foundation for Unintended Consequences *JAMA.* 2012;308(3):241-244.
113. Vennix JAM. *Group model building: facilitating team learning using system dynamics.* Chichester: John Wiley & Sons; 1996
114. Dangerfield B. System Dynamics applications to European health care issues. *Journal of the Operational Research Society.*50:345-353.
115. Elf M, Putilova, Mariya, von Koch, Lena , Öhrn, Kerstin. Using system dynamics for collaborative design: a case study. *BMC Health Services Research.* 2007;7:123.
116. Royston G DA, Townshend JP, and Turner H Using System Dynamics to help develop and implement policies and programmes in health care in England *System Dynamics Review.* 1999;15(3):293-313.
117. Abo-Hamad W, Rashwan, W., & Arisha, A. A system dynamics view of the acute bed blockage problem in the Irish healthcare system. *European Journal of Operational Research.* 2015;24(1):276-293.
118. Morath J. Nurses Create a Culture of Patient Safety: It Takes More Than Projects. *OJIN: The Online Journal of Issues in Nursing.* 2011;16(3).

119. n.a. *Pharmaceutical Industry Is Biggest Defrauder of the Federal Government under the False Claims Act, New Public Citizen Study Finds.* 1600 20th Street NW, Washington, D.C. 20009: Public Citizen;2010.
120. Knowx R. U.S. Ranks Below 16 Other Rich Countries In Health Report [Internet]. Washington DC: National Public Radio (NPR); 2013. Podcast: 3:23. Available from: http://www.npr.org/sections/health-shots/2013/01/09/168976602/u-s-ranks-below-16-other-rich-countries-in-health-report
121. Allen M. How Many Die From Medical Mistakes In U.S. Hospitals? [Internet]. Washington DC: National Public Radio (NPR); 2013. Podcast. Available from: http://www.npr.org/sections/health-shots/2013/09/20/224507654/how-many-die-from-medical-mistakes-in-u-s-hospitals?ft=1&f=1128
122. Curtin MA. *Quality Improvement, Patient Safety & Efficiency in Outpatient Practice* 221 Michigan St. NE, Suite 403 Grand Rapids, MI: MPIE Risk Management;2011.
123. Prentice JC, Pizer, Steven D. Delayed Access to Health Care and Mortality. *Health Serv Res* 2007;42(2):644-662.
124. Braun W. The System Archetypes: The Systems Modeling Workbook. http://wwwu.uniklu.ac.at/gossimit/pap/sd/wb_sysarch.pdf2002.
125. Sampson R, Morenoff, JD, Gannon-Rowley, T. L., Beauchamp, R. R., Faden, R. J. Assessing "neighborhood effects": social processes and new directions in research. *Annual Review of Sociology.* 2002;28:443-478.
126. Fisher ES WJ. Health care quality, geographic variations, and the challenge of supply-sensitive care. *Perspectives in Biology and Medicine.* 2003;46:69-79.
127. DHHS. Fact Sheet: The Opioid Epidemic By the Numbers. In: (DHHS) DoHaHS, ed. Washington DC: Department of Health and Human Services (DHHS); 2016.
128. Martin L LM, Hyatt J, Krueger J. *Addressing the Opioid Crisis in the United States.* Cambridge, Massachusetts: Institute for Healthcare Improvement (IHI);2016.
129. Martin L, Laderman A Systems Approach Is The Only Way To Address The Opioid Crisis, . *Health Affairs Blog.* 7500 Old Georgetown Road, Suite 600, Bethesda, MD 20814-6133: Health Affairs Blog; 2016.
130. Churchman CW. *The Systems Approach.* New York City: Dell; 1979.
131. Churchman CW. *Challenge to Reason.* New York City: McGraw-Hill; 1968.
132. Richmond B. Systems Thinking/System Dynamics: Let's Just Get On With It. *System Dynamics Review* 1994;10(2-3):135-157.
133. Senge PF. *The Fifth Discipline: The Art & Practice of The Learning Organization (Revised Edition).* New York City: Doubleday; 2006.
134. JHSPH. *The Prescription Opioid Epidemic: An Evidence-Based Approach.* Johns Hopkins Bloomberg School of Public Health, Johns Hopkins Center for Drug Safety and Effectiveness, and Johns Hopkins Center for Injury Research and Policy Johns Hopkins University, Baltimore, Maryland;2015.
135. CDC. Social Determinants of Health. *Healthy People 2020* 2016; https://www.healthypeople.gov/2020/topics-objectives/topic/social-determinants-of-health.
136. Schrag J. *The Social Determinants of Health: Homelessness and Unemployment.* 401 Ninth St. NW, Suite 900, Washington, DC 20004: America's Essential Hospitals;2014.

137. Hwang SW HM. *Health Care Utilization in Homeless People: Translating Research into Policy and Practice.* Washington, DC: Agency for Healthcare Research and Quality (AHRQ);2010.
138. Salit S.A. KEM, Hartz A.J., Vu J.M., Mosso A.L. Hospitalization costs associated with homelessness in New York City. *New England Journal of Medicine* 1998;338:1734-1740.
139. Martell J.V. SRS, Harada J.K., Kobayashi J., Sasaki V.K., Wong C. Hospitalization in an urban homeless population: the Honolulu Urban Homeless Project. *Annals of Internal Medicine.* 1992;116:299-303.
140. Rosenheck R SC. Homelessness: health service use and related costs. *Jounral of Med Care.* 1998;36(8):1121-1122.
141. n.a. *Cost of Homelessness, National Alliance to End Homelessness.* 1518 K Street NW, 2nd Floor, Washington, DC 20005: National Alliance to End Homelessness;2011.
142. Associates A. *Costs Associated With First-Time Homelessness For Families and Individuals.* Washington, DC: U.S. Department of Housing and Urban Developmen; 2010.
143. Stroh DP, Goodman, Michael. A Systemic Approach to Ending Homelessness. *Applied Systems Thinking Journal.* 2007;4.
144. Rwashana AS, Nakubulwa, Sarah, Nakakeeto-Kijjambu, Margaret, Adam, Taghreed Advancing The Application Of Systems Thinking In Health: Understanding The Dynamics Of Neonatal Mortality In Uganda. *Health Research Policy and Systems.* 2014;12(36):1478-4505.
145. n.a. *Committing to Child Survival: A Promise Renewed.* United Nations Children's Fund Unicef;2015.
146. Sterman JD. Learning from Evidence in a Complex World. *Am J Public Health* 2006;96(3):505-514.
147. Valentine A, Wexler, Adam, Kates, Jennifer *The U.S. Global Health Budget: Analysis of the Fiscal Year 2017 Budget Request.* Washington DC: Kaiser Family Foundation (KFF);2016.
148. Swanson C. What is Systems Thinking for Health. 2014; https://st4chealth.com/, 2016.
149. Katz R, Kornblet, Sarah, Arnold, Grace, Lief, Eric, Fischer, Julie E. Defining Health Diplomacy: Changing Demands in the Era of Globalization. *The Milbank Quarterly.* 2011;89(3):503–523.
150. NCI. *Using Systems Thinking and Tools to Solve Public Health Problems.* Washington DC, USA: National Cancer Institute (NCI); 2012.
151. Leischow SJ, Best, Allan, Trochim, William M., Clark, Pamela I., Gallagher, Richard S., Marcus, Stephen E., Matthews, Eva. Systems Thinking to Improve the Public's Health. *Am J Prev Med* 2008;35(2):196-203.
152. Smith M, Saunders, Robert, Stuckhard, Leigh, McGinness, J. Michael. *Best Care at Best Care at Lower Cost, The Path to Continuously Learning.* Washington DC: The National Academies Press; 2012.
153. Stefl M. *Futurescan: Healthcare Trends and Implications 2012–2017*: Health Administration Press (HAP); 2012.
154. Trochim W, Cabrera,DA, Milstein,B, Gallagher,RS and Leischow, SJ. Practical Challenges of Systems Thinking and Modeling in Public Health. *American Journal of Public Health.* 2006.

155. Frazer J, Fuster, Valentin. *GLOBAL HEALTH AND THE FUTURE ROLE OF THE UNITED STATES*. 500 Fifth Street, NW Washington, DC 20001: National Academies of Press (NAP) Science, Engineering and Medicine; 2017.
156. Ackoff RL. *Ackoff's Best: His Classic Writings on Management*. New York City: Wiley; 1999.
157. Ackoff RL, Addison, Herbert J., Cary, Andrew. *Systems Thinking for Curious Managers With 40 New Management f–Laws*. Axminster, Devon, United Kingdom: Triarchy Press; 2010.
158. Johnson A. 100 Unintended Consequences of Obamacare. *National Review* 2013. www.nationalreview.com/article/359861/100--unintended--consequences--obamacare--andrew--johnson
159. Jutte DP, Miller, Jennifer L., Erickson, David J. Neighborhood Adversity, Child Health, and the Role for Community Development. *Pediatrics*. 2015;135(2).
160. RWJF. *A Systems Thinking Approach to the Social Determinants of Health (SDOH)*. Princeton, New Jersey: Robert Wood Johnson Foundation (RWJF);2010.
161. Solutions C. *Not Making the Grade*. Oakland, CA: Robert Wood Johnson Foundation (RWJF);2014.
162. Thies KM. Identifying the educational implications of chronic illness in school children. *Journal of School Health*. 1999;69 (10):392-397.
163. Levine S. Psychological and social aspects of resilience: a synthesis of risks and resources *Dialogues in Clinical Neuroscience*. 2003;5(3):273-280.
164. Bisognano M KC. *Pursuing the Triple Aim: Seven Innovators Show the Way to Better Care, Better Health, and Lower Costs*. San Francisco: Jossey-Bass Publishers; 2012.
165. IHI. Institute for Healthcare Improvement (IHI). 2015; http://www.ihi.org/Pages/default.aspx.
166. Berwick DM, Nolan TW, Whittington J. The triple aim: care, health, and cost. *Health Aff (Millwood)*. 2008;27(3):759-769.
167. Kindig DA. Unpacking the Triple Aim Model. *Improving Population Health: Policy. Practice. Research.* Wisconsin: University of Wisconsin Department of Population Health Sciences; 2011.
168. Lewis N. Populations, Population Health, and the Evolution of Population Management: Making Sense of the Terminology in US Health Care Today. *Institute for Healthcare Improvement (IHI)*. MA: IHI; 2014.
169. NPS. *National Prevention Strategy (NPS)*. Washington, DC:: U.S. Department of Health and Human Services;2011.
170. James J. A New, Evidence – Based Estimate of Patient Harms Associated with Hospital Care. *Journal of Patient Safety*. 2013;9(3):122 – 128.
171. Levinson D. *Adverse Events in Skilled Nursing Facilities: National Incidence among Medicare Beneficiaries*. Washington DC: Department of Health and Human Services;2014.
172. Chassin MR, Loeb, . High-Reliability Health Care: Getting There from Here. *The Milbank Quarterly*. 2013;91(3):459-490.
173. AHRQ. High Reliability. *PSNET: Patient Safety Net*. 2016. https://psnet.ahrq.gov/primers/primer/31/high-reliability.
174. Schyve PM. Systems Thinking and Patient Safety. Vol 2. Advances in Patient S9afety ed: Agency for Healthcare Research and Quality (AHRQ); 2005.

175. AHRQ. Patient Safety Primer: High Reliability. *PSNet* 2016; https://psnet.ahrq.gov/primers/primer/31.
176. Griffith JR. Understanding High Reliability: Are Baldrige Recipeint Models? *Journal of Healthcare Management (JHM)*. 2015;60(1):44-61.
177. Pronovost P, Ravitiz, Alan, Grant, Conrad. How Systems Engineering Can Help Fix Health Care. *Harvard Business Review (HBR)*. 2017. https://hbr.org/2017/02/how-systems-engineering-can-help-fix-health-care.
178. Kenagy J. *Designed to Adapt: Leading Healthcare in Challenging Times.* 26 Shawnee Way C, Bozeman, MT: Second River Healthcare Pres; 2009.
179. Jenks SF, Williams, Mark V., Coleman, Eric A. Rehospitalizations among Patients in the Medicare Fee-for-Service Program. *N Engl J Med 2009; 360:1418-1428.* 2009;360:1418-1428.
180. Gleckman H. Preventing Hospital Readmissions. Howard Gleckman; 2011.

Index

accountable care organization, 133
Actors, vii, 63, 103, 107, 108
Affordable Care Act, 41, 144
Agency for Healthcare Research and Quality, 110, 164, 165
Agent-based modeling, 49, 53
applications, viii, ix, x, 2, 16, 100, 121, 132, 138, 139, 150, 151, 161, 162
Archetypes, 51, 52, 76, 77, 80, 81, 97, 142, 163
balancing feedback, 4, 28, 77, 79, 119, 120
boundaries, 5, 18, 24, 25, 35, 37, 48, 54, 100, 106, 124, 127, 128, 129, 132, 133, 134, 150
bounded rationality, 70
casual loops, x
Causal Loop Diagrams, iv, 50, 52, 73, 109, 111, 118, 119
Center for Disease Control and Prevention, 3, 106
Change management, 19
Chaos theory, 15
Chaotic systems, 16
closed systems, 13, 23, 25
collaboration, ix, 30, 37, 100, 115, 116, 124, 127, 132, 135
community, viii, ix, 2, 4, 5, 6, 7, 9, 10, 11, 12, 18, 24, 25, 26, 29, 31, 32, 33, 34, 35, 36, 40, 41, 42, 43, 45, 46, 47, 48, 51, 55, 63, 64, 65, 68, 75, 80, 81, 100, 101, 102, 103, 104, 105, 107, 108, 109, 111, 113, 115, 116, 119, 124, 126, 127, 128, 130, 132, 133, 134, 135, 136, 137, 138, 139, 140, 142, 148, 149
competencies, 40, 41, 100, 124, 126, 127, 128, 129, 133, 148, 149, 151
competency, ix, 3, 36, 130, 149, 150, 151
complex, viii, ix, x, 2, 3, 4, 5, 9, 11, 12, 15, 16, 17, 20, 21, 23, 24, 26, 27, 28, 29, 32, 33, 35, 38, 40, 41, 42, 43, 44, 45, 47, 48, 49, 50, 53, 54, 55, 57, 64, 65, 66, 68, 70, 71, 72, 73, 74, 75, 76, 77, 81, 97, 100, 105, 106, 110, 114, 118, 124, 126, 127, 128, 130, 131, 133, 135, 136, 139, 140, 142, 143, 148, 149, 150, 151, 161, 162
complex adaptive systems, 3, 15, 16, 26, 53
complexity, viii, x, 2, 3, 11, 12, 15, 16, 17, 22, 29, 32, 35, 36, 37, 38, 40, 41, 42, 44, 50, 52, 55, 63, 64, 65, 69, 70, 72, 74, 75, 77, 101, 106, 108, 117, 126, 128, 131, 132, 133, 140, 142, 143, 144, 149, 151, 158, 159
Complexity theory, 16
connections, 5, 11, 18, 22, 24, 38, 53, 57, 100, 132, 133
Continuous Learning Systems, 24
continuous quality improvement, 78, 101, 130, 142
Critical Success Factors, vii, 30
Cybernetics, 17, 158, 162
delays, 4, 10, 16, 40, 41, 50, 64, 65, 68, 69, 71, 73, 78, 79, 113, 118, 162
Designed Systems, 23
dynamic system, 4, 23, 64
dysfunctions, ix, x, 7, 24, 40, 76, 77
Ego-centric networks, 18
feedback, viii, 2, 4, 6, 8, 10, 16, 17, 19, 21, 23, 25, 28, 32, 35, 36, 40, 41, 42, 43, 50, 52, 58, 61, 62, 63, 64, 65, 66, 67, 68, 70, 71, 72, 73, 74, 77, 78, 79, 81, 118, 119, 121, 129, 139, 142, 143, 144, 146, 150, 151
feedback loops, viii, 2, 4, 8, 16, 17, 21, 23, 28, 32, 36, 40, 41, 42, 43, 50, 51, 52, 58, 61, 63, 64, 65, 66, 67, 68, 70, 71, 72, 73, 74, 79, 81, 105, 119, 120, 121, 139, 142, 143, 144, 151
flow chart, 53
flows, 17, 21, 35, 50, 53, 57, 58, 59, 64, 65, 71, 72, 74
Global health, 37, 38, 124, 128, 129
Health Leadership Alliance, 150
health systems, viii, ix, x, 2, 3, 5, 7, 9, 12, 13, 15, 17, 18, 23, 25, 26, 27, 29, 31, 32, 36, 37, 38, 40, 41, 42, 43, 47, 50, 53, 61, 64, 65, 72, 73, 74, 75, 76, 77, 100, 101, 102, 105, 108, 117, 124, 125, 126, 127, 128, 129, 132, 135, 139, 140, 142, 143, 146, 147, 148, 149, 150, 151, 155
healthcare system, 8, 10, 35, 160, 162

167

Healthy People 2020, vi, 109, 128, 137, 163
Homelessness, vi, 109, 110, 112, 114, 115, 163, 164
Information and communication theory, 18
Institute of Healthcare Improvement, 101
integrate, 3, 24, 79, 141, 149, 151
integration, ix, 2, 10, 12, 26, 38, 40, 41, 42, 43, 49, 55, 101, 104, 124, 125, 130, 134, 135, 137, 138, 139, 140, 144
interactions, viii, 4, 5, 8, 12, 15, 16, 17, 18, 21, 22, 23, 24, 26, 27, 29, 32, 35, 36, 38, 47, 49, 50, 55, 61, 70, 72, 100, 102, 118, 119, 121, 126, 129, 130, 131, 134, 142, 149
interconnected, ix, 2, 3, 5, 6, 9, 10, 13, 15, 22, 32, 35, 38, 40, 50, 55, 74, 108, 124, 126, 127, 128, 142, 144, 148, 149
interconnections, 3, 55, 134, 146
interdependence, 2, 9, 34, 38, 55, 124, 128, 129, 133, 149, 150, 151
interdependencies, viii, 2, 3, 32, 33, 42, 55, 60, 130, 133
interrelationships, 4, 5, 10, 42, 105, 118, 124, 132, 133, 136, 149
interventions, 10, 16, 17, 18, 27, 30, 31, 35, 36, 40, 48, 52, 53, 54, 63, 74, 101, 106, 107, 114, 115, 135, 139
leader development, 124, 127, 128, 151, 156
leaders, viii, ix, x, 2, 3, 4, 5, 9, 10, 11, 12, 18, 20, 21, 22, 26, 27, 31, 33, 35, 36, 38, 40, 41, 42, 43, 44, 46, 47, 48, 51, 52, 53, 54, 55, 58, 59, 63, 65, 68, 73, 76, 77, 79, 97, 100, 101, 102, 105, 106, 107, 108, 109, 111, 113, 116, 124, 126, 127, 128, 130, 131, 132, 133, 134, 135, 136, 137, 139, 140, 143, 144, 146, 147, 148, 149, 150, 151, 156, 158, 159
leadership, viii, ix, 2, 15, 22, 24, 34, 35, 40, 41, 43, 64, 76, 81, 124, 125, 127, 129, 130, 133, 134, 140, 142, 148, 156, 158, 159
limits to growth, 4, 144
linear processes, 105
methods, viii, ix, x, 2, 4, 11, 16, 17, 18, 40, 47, 48, 49, 51, 53, 54, 64, 65, 72, 75, 100, 101, 102, 117, 133, 142, 144, 148, 149, 151, 161
Natural Systems, 23
networks, 2, 17, 18, 26, 29, 32, 35, 36, 38, 40, 49, 53, 63, 65, 81, 105, 128
non-linear, viii, 2, 4, 16, 40, 41, 50, 57, 65, 74, 117, 148
Open Systems, 24
organizations, ix, x, 3, 4, 5, 7, 9, 10, 11, 12, 13, 15, 17, 18, 20, 22, 24, 25, 29, 32, 33, 34, 35, 36, 37, 38, 40, 46, 47, 48, 49, 51, 52, 53, 54, 55, 63, 64, 70, 74, 76, 80, 81, 100, 101, 104, 107, 112, 124, 126, 127, 128, 130, 131, 132, 134, 136, 137, 139, 140, 142, 143, 144, 146, 147, 148, 150, 151, 155, 156
patient-centered medical home, 55, 79, 115
patterns, 4, 5, 10, 11, 12, 14, 17, 19, 26, 27, 41, 47, 49, 51, 52, 53, 55, 68, 76, 97, 105, 107, 124, 129, 132, 133, 136, 139, 140, 161
planning, 10, 18, 21, 32, 49, 50, 52, 54, 72, 97, 101, 113, 132, 133, 134, 143, 151, 160
policies, 4, 9, 10, 16, 17, 21, 22, 23, 27, 33, 35, 36, 37, 40, 41, 49, 50, 51, 55, 64, 65, 71, 72, 73, 74, 75, 76, 77, 79, 103, 107, 130, 140, 156, 162
policy, viii, ix, x, 4, 5, 8, 9, 10, 17, 18, 19, 20, 27, 30, 32, 36, 37, 38, 40, 41, 42, 43, 48, 50, 51, 52, 54, 55, 58, 59, 63, 64, 67, 68, 71, 72, 74, 76, 79, 81, 100, 101, 102, 111, 126, 127, 129, 132, 133, 138, 142, 148, 149, 151, 155, 156
processes, 4, 9, 10, 11, 12, 16, 17, 20, 21, 22, 23, 24, 25, 27, 31, 33, 34, 35, 40, 42, 43, 44, 47, 49, 51, 53, 55, 56, 58, 61, 62, 63, 64, 71, 72, 73, 74, 76, 97, 100, 104, 105, 108, 129, 130, 132, 133, 139, 142, 143, 144, 150, 163
public health, viii, x, 4, 5, 7, 9, 12, 13, 16, 19, 24, 29, 30, 33, 34, 37, 40, 41, 42, 45, 46, 49, 50, 52, 53, 54, 58, 64, 75, 101, 104, 108, 124, 128, 129, 132, 133, 135, 139, 140, 149, 150, 161
Quadruple Aim, vi, 135, 137, 138, 139
Reductionism, 13

reinforcing feedback, 4, 51, 67, 78, 105
relationships, 4, 12, 15, 17, 18, 22, 32, 40, 47, 48, 49, 50, 52, 55, 60, 64, 65, 66, 70, 71, 72, 74, 106, 107, 118, 119, 124, 129, 130, 131, 142, 149
shared understanding, 11, 110
skills, ix, 34, 70, 74, 113, 128, 129, 133, 148
social determinants of health, 5, 9, 20, 24, 27, 30, 31, 33, 38, 40, 44, 64, 65, 100, 109, 124, 127, 128, 130, 134, 135, 137, 139, 140, 150
social network analysis, 16, 17, 160
Social network theory, 18
Socio-centric networks, 18
solutions, viii, ix, 2, 3, 4, 5, 9, 11, 22, 27, 33, 37, 38, 40, 46, 47, 48, 49, 50, 53, 54, 55, 63, 73, 75, 76, 77, 80, 97, 100, 101, 102, 106, 107, 108, 112, 113, 114, 116, 117, 124, 127, 128, 129, 130, 131, 134, 135, 140, 141, 142, 148, 149, 150
stakeholders, 2, 5, 10, 11, 17, 26, 32, 36, 38, 41, 42, 49, 50, 53, 63, 64, 75, 100, 101, 102, 105, 106, 107, 108, 111, 116, 118, 119, 121, 128, 130, 132, 134, 135, 136, 139, 140, 144, 150
stocks, 17, 21, 35, 50, 51, 52, 58, 59, 64, 65, 71, 74
strategic leader, 132, 133
subsystem, 7, 20, 23, 28, 35, 45, 100
sub-systems, 10, 20, 27, 40
subsystems, 6, 7, 8, 21, 22, 23, 24, 31, 35, 50, 77, 133, 146
system dynamics, 10, 16, 17, 27, 50, 64, 65, 72, 74, 75, 81, 111, 113, 118, 128, 135, 142, 148, 162
systemigram, 50
systems analysis, 5, 47, 48, 54
systems approach, ix, 5, 10, 32, 34, 37, 38, 40, 43, 46, 47, 48, 52, 54, 55, 100, 102, 108, 127, 135, 139, 141, 142, 143, 144, 147
systems dynamics, ix, x, 41, 50, 51, 52, 54, 64, 67, 68, 71, 100, 120, 124, 132, 140
systems science, 14, 151
Systems theories, 12, 20, 31
Systems Theory, 13, 14, 139, 158
systems thinking, viii, ix, x, 2, 3, 4, 5, 6, 8, 9, 10, 11, 12, 16, 17, 21, 22, 25, 26, 27, 29, 30, 34, 35, 36, 38, 40, 41, 45, 46, 47, 48, 49, 52, 53, 54, 55, 57, 63, 64, 65, 67, 68, 100, 101, 102, 105, 107, 108, 111, 116, 117, 118, 121, 124, 125, 126, 127, 128, 129, 130, 131, 132, 133, 134, 136, 140, 142, 143, 144, 146, 147, 148, 149, 150, 151, 155, 157, 160, 161
Systems Thinking for Health Strengthening, 150
Theoretical Biology, 14, 15
tools, viii, ix, x, 2, 4, 11, 34, 35, 40, 46, 47, 48, 49, 50, 51, 52, 53, 54, 64, 65, 72, 100, 101, 102, 111, 117, 127, 132, 139, 142, 148, 149, 151, 162
Triple Aim, vi, x, 5, 9, 27, 40, 41, 43, 135, 136, 137, 138, 139, 140, 165
Uganda, vi, 117, 118, 120, 121, 164
unintended consequence, 81, 113
unintended consequences, 9, 10, 17, 20, 24, 26, 40, 48, 51, 64, 65, 69, 74, 76, 80, 81, 102, 126, 127, 129, 131, 133, 146, 148, 149, 162
Veteran's Affairs, 79
World Health Organization, 3, 4, 29, 65, 127, 129, 137, 150, 155, 157, 160, 162

Made in the USA
Middletown, DE
15 June 2021

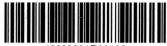